MW01716451

Life and Times of Sadie

Snacks & Attacks

By

Sandy Lockwood

Table of Contents

Dedication

This book is dedicated to my mom. Your love was unconditional. Your protection was fierce. Your drive and strength were undeniable. Thank you for making the sacrifices you did.

Acknowledgement

I would like to acknowledge everyone who has been traumatized or abused. If you have ever felt small, helpless, voiceless, or unseen, I see you. I have left out so many details because I want to respect the story that is not mine to tell. While this is a watered down version of events, it is by no means a laugh in the face of abuse. I hope every victim of abuse gets the help they need in order to heal and find peace.

Thank you to all of my friends and family that have been encouraging and supportive.

A special thanks to Candy and Amber. Candy, you have been more supportive than a 1955 brassierre. I know some of this process has not be easy or fun. You lived the paragraphs that weren't written and I know this journey wasn't always comfortable. Amber, thank you for always being up for a good adventure. I appreciate all of the time you took out of your day to take 92749 pics. The author pic and cover photo are perfect.

Last but never least, my momma. You always believed in me. You bought me a word processor as an investment into my writing future when I was very young. It took awhile but I finally put something out there for the world to read. I hope I respected your story while telling mine.

About the Author

Sandy is a 51 year old self proclaimed free spirit. She lives in West Texas with her husband, 2 dogs, 2 Norwegian Dwarf goats, and a Flemish Giant rabbit. She has 2 sons, a daughter-in-law, and a grand daughter.

Sandy has always loved writing and aspired to become a published writer. She was always very self conscious of her writings and never shared them. When Covid took over, and people were taking to social media to entertain themselves and their loved ones by sharing their talent or passion, Sandy started sharing her stories. After a lot of positive feedback, love, and support, she started writing her first book.

Sandy loves spending time with her family and taking care of her animals. She has recently become a new grandmother and enjoys every second she gets with her grand baby. Daily farm chores and household chores keep her busy, but she always finds time for meditation, journaling, being a medical advocate for her friends and family, and cheering at local softball games.

Sandy and her husband bought a camper and have officially become happy campers. This is their newest passion. There is nothing that seems to center them more than a weekend at a State Park filled with hiking, playing cards, star gazing, and a nice camp fire with no cell service.

There are a few things you can always count on when Sandy is around...Snacks and Shenanigans.

INTRODUCTION

It was a cold, icy January in 1972. My mother was 3 weeks from her due date with me when she awoke to contractions. My dad was a bit of a partier and had the roaming eye (not to mention other roaming parts). It was not yet daybreak, and he was just dragging in from a night of debauchery. He was, what we in the south call, drunker than Cooter Brown. There is no way he would be able to drive my mom to the hospital or be responsible enough to be left with my older sister, Katie, who was 2 at the time.

This is where the dilemma starts. My mom needed to get to the hospital. She could not call her mother for a ride because her mom, my nanny, was not a fan of my dad. With his drinking came a lot of aggressive, abusive, and controlling behavior. My mom tried to keep that tightly tucked in, but it was hard to hide black eyes. If my nanny would have come over, it would have ended up in a big brawl. She would not want a drunken fool in the room when her grandbaby was born. She damn sure would not have wanted to ride in the same vehicle with him or leave Katie with him. My dad would not want my Nanny driving off with my mom because, well, that was his wife and his property. He couldn't afford to have her alone with anyone who may tell her that she didn't have to live this way.

My dad's mom, my Mawmaw, would not be an option as she did not drive. My pawpaw was driving the family home from church one Sunday morning when an oilfield truck came roaring down the road and hit them head on. My pawpaw sustained significant injuries, while my Mawmaw had non-life-threatening injuries. My dad was in the backseat and was holding his 18-month-old brother. They were both thrown from the vehicle, and the baby died. Some say this is what caused my dad's erratic behavior, the head injury he sustained, along with the death of his brother. Anywho, my Mawmaw never drove and rarely ever got in a vehicle after that accident.

By this time, my mother is sure that she will deliver at home. She is panicked as to how she will get to the hospital safely. She had several miscarriages and a baby that passed away 6 weeks after birth. The fact that she is in labor 3 weeks early with no ride to the hospital is causing a lot of stress.

My dad has a brother that is much younger than him. He was 15 years old. He does not have a driver's license and has never driven on icy roads or the highway. That was the brilliant idea my dad had, though. He called his brother and told him to load up Mawmaw and head on over to pick him and my mom up. My mom quickly packed a bag and called my nanny. She told her that she had awoken suddenly with contractions and was going to the hospital. My mom assured her that she was ok and would feel so much better if she knew Katie was being cared for while she was gone. Katie would be going to Nanny's.

Ok, done deal. Everything is settled. Katie is dropped off, and the trek to the hospital has begun. Did I mention the hospital is in a little town about 15-20 minutes away? And the roads are icy? And a 15 yrs. old inexperienced and unlicensed boy is driving? This is where it gets interesting. Mawmaw is in the back seat with my mom. She is trying to focus on the impending birth and not on the car sliding all over the road. She has severe anxiety when it comes to riding in cars, and even the laboring daughter-in-law cannot distract her from that. She screams and prays as they drive. My dad is being the drunken boss and giving directions and lectures. Anytime there is a mistake made, his brother gets a slap to the back of the head. That only makes him more nervous and, in turn, his driving worse. That makes the screams more frequent and the prayers a bit more urgent. My mom is the only calm one at this point.

They finally arrive at the hospital. My mom was quickly taken into the delivery room and promptly gave birth to a 5-pound, 2-ounce baby girl. That would be me, Sadie Sue. That would also be the first and last time I was ever listed as underweight.

CHAPTER 1

Hi. My name is Sadie Sue. There are a few things you should know about me before I go any further. I grew up in the 70s in a small, West Texas oilfield town. The economy solely relies on the oilfield. When the oil market is good, the town thrives. People move in by the droves. All other businesses in town lose employees to the oilfield, housing prices go up, and makeshift housing is seen in the form of tents and RVs. They call it a boom. When the market isn't doing well, the town shrivels up, people lose their jobs and move, crime goes up, homelessness increases, and businesses close. They call this a bust. The rest of life in this small town is dictated by religion and politics. It's not like you have a choice in either, you are Christian, and you are Republican.

My mom and dad divorced when I was 2. My mom worked 2 full-time jobs and mowed lawns in her spare time. Seriously, she called it spare time. My sister and I would walk to school and usually walk home. We were called latch key kids. I am not sure who coined the phrase, but it was a name given to the kids who walked home and used a key to let themselves in the house. The 70s were sort of revolutionary for women. They were starting to be seen as independent and not known as property. They were no longer tolerating abuse and were leaving their marriages in the dust. They were making their name in the workforce and supporting themselves. Everything wasn't roses, by any means. Women still made significantly lower wages than men and had to put up with what is now known as sexual harassment in the workplace. The system did not back these women. The mentality was that you left a perfectly fine home and chose to do this, so, do it. Child support was laughable. It did not deter these women. Off to work they went and off to walking to and from school their kids went.

My mom, sister, and I lived with my grandparents until my mom saved enough money for a downpayment on a house. Our house was built 2 blocks behind my grandparents' house. We would walk back and forth between the houses. It was not uncommon for us to show up at my Nanny's house telling her we had not eaten, and we only had cereal at home. Nanny always had a nice, hot, home cooked meal on the table. She would have gladly fed us every night even if we didn't tell her the cereal bluff. The funny thing is our dog, Tiny, caught on and would run to Nanny's when she got in trouble or just wanted table scraps instead of canned dog food.

My mom's parents, Nanny and Gramps, were the story book grandparent's. Gramps was a Marine who had fought in WWII. After he left the Marines, he took a job as a geologist in the oilfield. Nanny was a nurse. She worked in a doctor's office Monday through Friday. She worked in a little town about 15-20 miles away. She would normally get home around 6 pm, and then she would start cooking. My gramps was very old school and had to have a home cooked meal with the table set at a certain time. He was very regimented, and she was not. She always cooked and always had a homemade cake on the counter. She kept a plethora of crafts for us and let us put on elaborate plays in her living room. She had the patience of a highly medicated sloth.

Gramps, on the other hand, was not known for his patience. He traveled a lot for his job and was rarely home. The house was our giant playground when he was gone. When he was home, she would ask us to behave while he was there. We tried, but it usually did not work out well for me. He was not abusive. He never spanked us. He would scratch his head and grumble. Nanny would always smile and present us with some new craft project to keep us quiet and out of his hair. It was especially necessary to keep us out of the way when the Cowboys were playing football. He was a diehard fan, and nothing could interrupt his time watching the games.

My other set of grandparents was very different. Different does not mean bad. It was just different. My Pawpaw owned a local gas station, and my Mawmaw would iron clothes for people to earn extra money. Neither of them was regimented. There was no schedule. You would go to bed when you wanted, and you would wake up when you wanted. Both of my grandmothers were night owls, and I loved it. My Mawmaw did not cook a large meal at a certain time, nor did she set a traditional table. If you wanted a burger, she cooked you a burger. It didn't matter if it was 1 pm or 8 pm. I really like that. There were no crafts and no homemade cakes. There was a large bucket on the counter filled with all kinds of goodies from the day-old bread store. Once it expired, it went to the day-old bread store (that was really the name of the store), and you could get a huge bargain on snacks. The counter was also lined with every flavor of soda. This is the place I liked to be when I was feeling a bit nervous. The possibilities were endless for gluttony.

She did not drive, so we didn't have outings with her like we did with Nanny. With Mawmaw, we sat at her big dining room table and talked. She would have a cup of coffee, a cigarette, and all of the local gossip. For a kid that never sat still, I could sit and listen to her for hours.

There were no cell phones, ring doorbells, security cameras, or GPS tracking. When we woke up on the weekends, we were expected to go outside and play all day. You didn't come home until it started getting dark and the streetlights came on. Video games were not even a factor. Atari came out in 1977. This meant a good portion of my time was spent outside, unsupervised.

My sister, Katie, was the older sister. She took her role very seriously. She was the boss, and she doled out the rules and responsibilities. She didn't like to be dirty, and she didn't like to play outside. Most of her free time was spent playing with her Barbies. I could have sworn it was mainly spent making new rules for me. Katie was the one that had a plan for emergencies. Like an actual plan. She would also be the one who tried to talk sensibly to adults who were fussing. She looked for a resolution or tried to bargain to deescalate a situation.

I was the opposite of Katie. I was loud. I loved being outside. I hated Barbies. I also hated rules. There was no such thing as ADHD at the time, or I would have been heavily medicated. I talked a lot. I moved a lot. I stayed up all night. My mind was full of information, questions, and scenarios at all times. I loved to make people laugh. It was one of my coping skills. If I could feel any sort of tension, I would do something ridiculous to get a laugh. Katie swore that I just wanted to be the center of attention. It was my way of breaking the tension and lightening the mood. By all means, look at me and laugh at me if it means that no one is going to be upset or have a raised voice. My other coping skill, snacks. After the laughs faded and situations were avoided, and sometimes after the shit hit the fan, you could find me eating. This meant I often had a bellyache. My belly either hurt because I was stressed and nervous, or it hurt because I had just hidden away somewhere and eaten 4 honey buns and slammed two coca colas.

It was not uncommon for me to hold in all of my emotions. No one knew if I was scared, nervous, worried, or upset. I looked like the happiest, funniest kid around. The thing was, I could only hold all those feelings in for so long, then I would just lose it. The proverbial straw that broke the camel's back. I would have a crazy outburst. You would never expect to see or hear the things you would see or hear from me when I "lost my shit". I can laugh about it now, but at the time, I felt like there was something really wrong with me. Of course, I would have to grab a snack and self soothe. I'm telling you, I was a hot mess of a kid.

One day, I was walking home from school by myself, minding my own business. I was in third grade and was at a new school because our house had just been built. I had my lunchbox in one hand and my notebook in the other. Three boys were walking behind me. They kept making fun of me and calling me names. I kept walking. I gave no response. They called me fat and laughed at me. I kept walking. They started kicking at my lunchbox and trying to knock my notebook out of my hand, all while laughing their little faces off. The ringleader was a big boy.

He was known as the school bully. He always had a few followers with him. I never liked him and always tried to steer clear of him. For whatever reason, today was the day he decided to press my buttons. I tried and tried to ignore him. I kept hoping the boys with him would decide that they weren't going to join in and be mean to him. I kept hoping they would tell him that he was being mean, and that he needed to stop. After blocks and blocks of no response from me, ol' bully boy decided to kick it up a notch and start saying things about my mom. Listen, you can call me fat all you want, but don't call my mom names. I felt my face getting hotter and hotter, my grip on my lunchbox and notebook were tighter and tighter, and my pace was faster and faster. My house would be just around the corner if I could just make it a few more steps. Right as I was approaching my street, Ol' Bully Boy kicked my notebook, and it went flying (I failed to mention I am a bit OCD and don't like my things out of order). I see my papers flying, and I hear him laugh and say my momma is a bitch. I turned around and started wailing on him with my lunchbox. He fell, and I started kicking him. If his little balls had dropped, they were now sitting snuggly next to his tonsils. The whole time I was screaming at him, 'Who is the BITCH now? You BITCH!". As quickly as it had happened, it stopped. I picked up my papers and my notebook, turned around, and walked home. I didn't say a word about it. Later that evening, his mother called my mom and told her that I had probably caused her poor, sweet son to be incapable of producing children. My mom got off the phone and told me what Ol' Bully Boy's mom had said and asked me if I had done that. I told her the story. I think she wanted me to apologize but knew she couldn't trust that I wouldn't call him a bitch in front of his mom. Just in case you are wondering, Ol' Bully Boy never bullied me again. If I had to guess, he probably went on to have children and lead a totally normal little bully life.

I cannot even fathom the load my mom carried on her shoulders or the stress she felt. She was a hard worker and kept a strict budget. She was a tiny, blonde with bright green eyes. She stood 5 feet tall and weighed approximately 98 pounds. She was not weak or frail. She had a very muscular build. She worked in the meat market. It was always deemed a man's world, and she was determined to work toe to toe with any man in the industry. And she did. She was known to be tough as a boot and extremely dependable. She never missed a day of work. It was common for her to get calls about my behavior or calls from myself or my sister me asking her to settle a fight we were having. She had a full plate and did not have time for the phone calls. My mom did not want to be seen as a woman in the workplace; she wanted to be seen as an equal. When the phone calls would come in, it took her away from work, and it also shined a light on her that said, 'MOM! LADY WORKING IN A MAN'S WORLD BUT HAVING TO TAKE TIME OUT OF THE WORK DAY FOR MOM STUFF'. She would beg us not to call and to behave so no one else called. Bless her heart, it never worked.

Years later, we had a 60th birthday party for my mom. All the butchers she had worked with showed up. They all told stories about how hard she worked and how strong she was. Of course, they could all recall a few stories about the phone calls. After all those years, they could remember very distinctly the fights Katie and I would have. There were times that my mom wouldn't get on the phone, and they had to hear our problems and relay the message to our mom. The best story of the night was a story about my mom fighting to be accepted as one of 'the guys' she worked with. She worked just as many hours and just as hard. She was dependable, and she knew the trade. She trained many of the butchers. She was not allowed to be a butcher because it was a man's job. Her title was meat wrapper. She excelled at that position and learned the butcher role as well.

All the guys would take a daily break at the same time. They would walk off and leave her in the market alone. She would often ask to join them, and they always said it was just the guys. That was pretty offensive to her. She worked alongside them and even trained some of them, yet she was not allowed to go to break with them. It didn't stop her from asking. Every day, she would ask to join them on break, and every day they would turn her down. She thought she would eventually wear them down. It never happened. I guess her anger and resentment grew every time she was rejected. As the story goes, it was an ordinary day. Break time came for the men, and they started to walk off. My mom started to walk off with them. They asked what she was doing and told her it was just the guys going on break. They say this tiny Nancy Sinatra look-alike whipped out a huge dildo from her coat pocket, threw it on the counter, and told them, "Here's my dick. Let’s go on break”. She was never ostracized from another break.

CHAPTER 2

As much as I hated schedules, I think they were good for me. During the time we lived with my Nanny, I do not remember being overly anxious. We woke up at a certain time, we ate at a certain time, bathed at a certain time, and had a bedtime. I think my Nanny did a great job at herding us out of the room when any discussion of my parent's divorce or the shenanigans that went along with it were being discussed. I felt like I was in a safe cocoon.

My mom had been working and saving to get us a home of our own. Finally, she had the money. She found a vacant lot 2 blocks behind my grandparents' house and started the ball rolling.

Everything seemed to be coming together. Life was moving in a positive direction, and my mom was crushing the goals she had set for herself.

While our home was being built, we moved into an apartment. This was the first time that I remembered being on our own. It felt a little scary to me. It made me feel very vulnerable. We lost the safety of my grandparents. I know now that they would not have been able to stop any tomfoolery that my dad may have caused, but at the time, they were my superheroes. My safety net was gone. Up until this point, I don't recall hoarding food or hiding to devour it. My weight was that of an average child my age.

Move in day started off with a bang. We pulled up to the apartment complex with the windows rolled down on the red cutlass supreme my mom had bought (another goal). There was a song on the radio that was about a party two doors down. I remember looking at our apartment from the car and looking down two doors. I wondered to myself if the people inside were laughing, drinking, and having a party. Enough daydreaming; time to climb out and start this new adventure. I pushed the white, bucket seat forward and hurled myself out of the car. We had an upstairs apartment. I stood in the parking lot and looked at the staircase and then let my eyes slowly look at the front door to my new home. My stomach hurt. Katie was dishing out orders.

She was in a hurry for me to gather a few things and get inside the apartment to look at our new room. She already had a plan for what went where. I would have my instructions as to what I could and could not touch soon. I gathered a few things and made my way up the stairs. I could still hear the music playing when I opened the front door to my new home. What I didn't know was that someone had opened the back door. The front door was about 20 feet directly in front of the back door. I tried to shuffle through the door with my load of goods for our bedroom, but the door was heavy and had a huge wind force behind it from. Because the other door was open, my door was being pulled shut. The next thing I knew, the door had slammed shut, and everything had made it to the other side safely except my finger. I stood there with one arm full of items and the other arm extended towards the door, and my index finger in between the door and door frame. I screamed. My mom and Katie came running. Mom opened the door, and my fingernail was standing up like a soldier standing at attention. Blood started to run down my hand. Mom was trying to assess the situation and calm me down. Katie was gathering up the things I had dropped and telling me that I had better not have gotten blood on any of her things. I hate it here. I hate that stupid song that is still playing. Can we go back to Nanny's? Can we at least go get a snack?

I would wander around the apartment complex and look for someone to chat with. One day, I happened to see the couple that lived below us. I made my way over and started to talk to them. They were an older couple. By the looks of her grey hair and his balding, their stooped posture, and slow, shuffling walk, I would say they were much older than my grandparents. I noticed they had small numbers tattooed on their wrists. This seemed very odd to me. Tattoos were very taboo back then, and the only people you saw with them were military men and bikers. This couple looked like neither of those. They felt very safe. They were very kind. I was never the kid that had a filter. What I was thinking often flew out of my mouth, much to my mom's dismay. I asked why they had tattoos and what they meant. Were they bikers? Were they in the military? They told me they were Jewish and had been in concentration camps. They were the first people I remember meeting that were not Christian.

From that point on, I found myself in their apartment a lot. She cooked Jewish foods and would save some for me. The latkes!! They would teach me their songs and play their games with me. I was pretty good at spinning the dreidel. Ok, maybe I spun the dreidel like it was a Tasmanian devil, but I had fun. They were so patient and loving. I could not imagine anyone being mean to them. It was the first time I realized that there were other people, good people, in the world who suffered at the hands of mean people.

My mom had decided to get a babysitter for us during the summer. We had never had a babysitter, and I was not fond of the idea. We were in an apartment complex, and my mom did not feel safe leaving us there alone while she was at work. She would interview teenage girls and grill them. She would give them all her requirements, and the ones that agreed would be hired. I had one boss, Katie, and I didn't need another one.

One of the girls had her boyfriend over and locked us out. She tricked us into going outside, and she shut and locked the door. One of the requirements was no boys or friends were allowed over, and they couldn't stay on the phone. My mom made it clear she was paying for someone to watch us. I was not happy about being locked out of my own home. I jumped from the porch, over the railing, onto the back porch. That hussy locked the sliding glass door! She didn't shut the curtain, though. I saw her making out with her boyfriend. I promptly jumped back onto the main stoop, marched myself down the stairs, and knocked on my neighbor's door. I told them I needed to use their phone to call my mom. Yep, another work phone call. Babysitter 1, down.

The next babysitter wanted to sit inside and talk on the phone. I could sit and talk to elderly people all day, but I could not sit and listen to a teenage girl talk to her boyfriend on the phone for 5 minutes. Not doing it! I wanted to go swimming. I repeated that phrase at least 9475 times.

She continued to ignore me. My mom had a list of chores for the babysitter. One of which was to vacuum. I unplugged the phone from the wall and reminded her that my mom did not pay her to talk on the phone. She rolled her eyes and told me to go get my swimsuit. While I was getting my swimsuit out, she got the vacuum cleaner out. She turned it on and promptly ran over my swimsuit. It sucked up into the vacuum and gave a whirl followed by a sputter as it died an agonizing death. Touché', Ms. Swimsuit Sucker Upper. Never one to backdown, I started taking the vacuum cleaner apart and trying to free my swimsuit. I finally got half of the suit freed, but it had large runs in the bottom and crotch from the tug of war. It was unwearable. She informed me we could not go swimming if I did not have a swimsuit. I went into my room and dug through all of the dresser drawers until I came out with a small bikini with lady bugs on it. I had spent a lot of time eating latkes with my new friends but had no idea my ladybug bikini would not fit.

Whether it was a good fit or not, I was going to shove myself in that swimsuit just to put a burr in the britches of Chatty Cathy. Yes, she was back on the phone. I jumped, tugged, and grunted until I had that suit on. I walked in the living room and announced it was time to swim. She looked at me and said, 'You are too big for that. You are too fat'. This was before the incident with Ol' Bully Boy, and I was shocked that I was called fat. I was so mad and so embarrassed. I cried. I cried as I grabbed some snacks and, went in my room, and inhaled them. Babysitter 2, down.

My mom had started seeing a man that she worked with. He was a nice guy. He loved my mom. His eyes sparkled when he looked at her. He had never been married and did not have kids. He was younger than my mom but assured her that he loved Katie and myself as his own. He really wanted to impress my mom. Everyone that knew my mom knew that her kids had to be happy. She didn't want us to feel left out or to ever be mistreated. Up to this point, she has had several first dates. This was the first guy that made it passed the first date and liked kids. When we had no babysitter, and my mom had to go to work, it seemed pretty normal that the new guy would volunteer. My mom tried to talk him out of it, but he insisted, and she needed to work. She gave him a rundown on us, the rules, and what to expect. I was pretty nervous about this situation. I liked this guy, but I wasn't sure I wanted to stay with him all day. I was a bit weary of men. My safe place was with kind, little women who liked to talk. This guy had always been nice to us, but my mom had always been there. Would he be nice if she wasn't there? He constantly told me I needed to be respectful and needed to say 'yes, ma'am' and 'no, ma'am' when speaking to my mother. He even wrote it in my autograph book! I didn't feel like I was disrespectful, but I had never been taught to use ma'am and sir. I wasn't sure how you just started doing that.

Because I was nervous, I had been eating my way through all the snacks. I even ate all the food my sweet, Jewish friend had baked. I was thinking up all sorts of scenarios and eating them away. The night before the big day of boyfriend babysitter, I had a bellyache. I kept telling my mom my stomach hurt, and I was crying and begging her not to go to work. She tried her best to soothe me. When that didn't work, she tried to be rational with me. She explained that she had to work, and she had to pay bills. Missing one day of work would leave her without enough money to cover our bills. She begged me to relax, get a good night's rest and, try to have fun tomorrow, and to behave. I heard that word a lot, BEHAVE.

I found some stowed away Easter candy and soothed myself.

The next day, the boyfriend came over. He was so excited. I never could figure out why he was so happy to watch two raggedy kids. Now that I am older, I know that he was seeing the brownie points rack up like a Vegas slot machine. He had a big, jacked up, bright orange truck. His plan was to keep us busy. Our first excursion was to wash the big truck. It wasn't that fun for us, but it was tolerable because he stopped to grab us some fast food before he went to the car wash. I didn't mind sitting in the truck, eating French fries and slurping on soda while he washed his truck. Katie, she was busy watching me. We were always together. She never yelled at the babysitters or pulled any shenanigans like I did. She watched and took mental notes. She would report every detail as if she were a private investigator, and our mom hired her. Occasionally, she would say, ‘I’m telling’ or ‘don’t say or do that to my sister’. Anywho, we got the truck washed, and I polished off my food and some of Katie’s before we returned to the apartment. As soon as we entered the apartment, the phone started ringing. It was for the boyfriend. His buddy was calling, asking him to meet at the arcade for a game of foosball. He got off the phone and gave us a hyped-up speech about how he was going to take us to an arcade, and we were going to have so much fun. Off we went.

We get to the arcade, and Boyfriend Babysitter sees his buddy right away. They start talking and walking over to the arcade machine they are going to play. It seems like there is a lot riding on this game because they are very serious. After they boast their game playing skills and make a friendly bet, Boyfriend Babysitter goes to the machine that takes your dollar and spits out 4 quarters. He ran a few dollars through the machine and handed Katie and me a handful of quarters. This was not my place. This was not my place at all. It was dark and musty. The carpet felt sticky. Each step I took was followed by a slight wrrrp when I lifted my shoe. There were so many lights flashing and so many sounds. Beeps, whirls, buzzing, and ringing were some of the sounds that were trying to be drowned out by blasting rock music. I walked over to the game Boyfriend Babysitter was playing and tugged on his arm. I told him I needed to go. He told me to let him finish this game. The sounds got louder. The lights became brighter. The carpet became stickier. I wanted to go. I tugged and tugged on his arm. He jerked his arm away and told me he was almost finished with this game. He said I couldn't tug on his arm or I would make him lose. He pointed me to the vending machines and told me to grab a snack. I walked over to the vending machine and used all my money for candy. Katie was at my side, telling me it would be ok. I did not feel like it was going to be ok. I walked back to the game Boyfriend Babysitter was playing and told him I didn't feel good. He gave me some more quarters and told me to grab a soda. I walked back to the machine and came back with an orange soda. I drank it at warp speed. Katie is holding my hand, repeating that everything is going to be ok. I started chanting, 'I don't feel good. I don't feel good'. Boyfriend Babysitter assured me his game was almost over.

He was talking very loudly and with a lot of enthusiasm. I'm not sure what game he was playing, but he was very invested. He was standing on one side of the machine and his friend on the other. They were each swatting at a roller ball while profusely sweating. I could feel the orange soda bubbling up in my throat. I was lifting my feet and feeling the wrrrp of the stickiness of the carpet. I looked around at the lights and listened to all the sounds. My head was spinning. I felt nauseous. My stomach was growling. I told my mom I didn't feel good last night, and here I am in an arcade feeling 12946 times worse. I said very loudly, 'I DON'T FEEL GOOD. I NEED TO GO HOME. I NEED TO GO HOME NOW!'. Boyfriend Babysitter never looked up. He just swatted at that roller ball, dropped some sweat on the table, and said he was winning. He was almost finished; he would win, and then we would leave. Katie chimed in and said she thought we needed to go.

I am not sure if he won or lost that game, but I do know he walked out of there as a total and completer loser. The last words I said to him were that I needed to use the bathroom, and then I started to cry. Katie started patting my back, and all of a sudden, I shit myself. The swatting noise stopped. It seemed like everything stopped. I think every noise stopped and the house lights came on. There I was, crying and standing in a pool of shit. Diarrhea, I might add. I mean, I had been complaining of a bellyache, all the while eating my misery away. What did they expect? Katie instinctively starts to tell me it is ok and usher me out the front door. Boyfriend Babysitter is stunned. He doesn't know what to do. He signed up to make brownie points with the love of his life, not to clean up a kid that shit herself in public. After we get outside, he realizes that he doesn't want me in his truck. I have liquid poo running down my legs and dripping on the floor. I can see the horror on his face, and it makes me cry louder and harder.

Katie is trying to find some paper towels (like that will help), and Boyfriend Babysitter is trying to hoist me into the bed of his truck. It was just enough movement to make me nauseous. At that moment, I puked.

It was a long ride home. I was sitting in the bed of a freshly washed truck, in a pool of diarrhea with vomit dangling from my hair. Katie was in the backseat but had the slider window open.

She kept telling me everything was ok and not to cry. On the way home, we pulled into the carwash. Boyfriend Babysitter sprayed the bed of his truck with the power hose and gave me a quick spray, too. It sure was much more fun the first go round when I was sitting inside with a happy meal. Babysitter 3, down.

CHAPTER 3

It was no secret that I did not handle change well. My mom thought if she put us in an activity that, it would help. She thought we would join some group, make friends, and have so much fun that we would transition into all the new things with ease. First, we had just left Nanny's and moved into an apartment. Then we had babysitters, and mom had a boyfriend. Soon we will be moving into our new house. We had never played sports or been in any out of school activity. Katie did not attend Kindergarten because our dad would not allow it. He wasn't the man of our house any longer; mom was. And she was making decisions.

I understand her thought process thus far. It gets a little sketchy for me from this point on. I was not a girly girl. I did not like to wear dresses, and if the truth be told, I didn't like to wash or brush my hair on most days. I didn't like the rules. I didn't like being without my sister. I was not athletic.

What activity or group could my mom possibly sign me up for? That was exactly the question I had. It was answered, but not with an answer I was hoping for. BROWNIES! Yes, you read that correctly. I was signed up for Brownies.

If you don't know what a Brownie is, it is the junior version of a Girl Scout. You wear a brown dress with a sash. You learn new things and participate in activities to earn badges that are sewn onto that sash. There are weekly meetings and sporadic outings. There is a code of conduct form that you have to read, and you and your parents have to sign it. You have monthly dues that your parents have to pay, and you have to sell cookies. Count me in for the cookie sales, but other than that, it's a no for me. She signed me up.

First order of business is to buy the uniform. There is one store in town that carries the Brownie/Girl Scout uniforms. It is a fancy schmancy store. We never shopped there because we could not afford it. It was such a pretty department store. It had a section for women's shoes, and they were displayed on brass tables with glass tops. There were glass cases that were beautifully lit up and held the latest perfume fragrances. The ceilings were high, and floors were carpeted in small sections and tiled in others. The click clack of high heeled shoes echoed throughout.

We walked in (no click clacking) and went to the small section dedicated to Brownie uniforms. Katie was in heaven. This was where she dreamt of shopping. She was looking around and taking in every sight, sound, and scent. I was dragging my feet and complaining. My mom started looking through the uniforms as a saleslady walked up. She asked if she could help, and mom told her what we were looking for and our sizes. I remember hearing Katie's size being slim, and then I hear my mom say that I needed a 6X or husky. What? husky? Am I husky? Why am I an X? I want to be slim. All of these things are running through my mind when I hear the saleslady say that they do not have anything in my size at this time. She can get Katie fixed up, and we will have to come back next week to get me squared away.

Obviously, they lost my attention. I immediately started looking for a place to hide. Lucky for me, they have big, round clothes racks scattered throughout the store. I run and run and finally pick a rack that appeals to my senses. In I go. My mom is now walking around the store with an arm draped with Brownie items while assertively calling my name. She was trying to be as forceful and as quiet as possible. We had already shown these shoppers more excitement than they had ever seen. When she would get near the rack I was hiding under, I would pop out and run until I found another suitable rack. In I would go. My middle name was now being added, and it was being said louder. I was hunkered down and about to run like a rabbit on the hunt... I hear my mom getting closer, and out I go. Except this time, I was not running. She had grabbed my arm. I tugged and pulled until I got loose and ran back into the rack. My mom was parting the clothes on that rack like Jesus parting the Red Sea. That didn't last long because the rack tumbled on its side. Whoopsey! Someone is getting a whoopin' tonight.

The saleslady called when my size came in. She was kind enough to hold my uniform at the sales counter. Mom didn't even have to walk to the back of the store and search for them. More importantly, she didn't have to bring me in with her. I am now officially a Brownie. I have my uniform, and I have my code of conduct form signed. I am going to my first meeting tonight.

I'm not sure what to call the ladies that are running this meeting. Are they teachers? Counselors? Big Brownies? They are talking in really high-pitched voices with their hands clasped in front of them. When they speak, they unclasp their hands, smile really big, say something in a tone that I am almost positive dolphins could hear, then clasp their hands. They seem nice but very theatrical. I have spotted a table to the side of the room that has refreshments. They can talk, clasp, and smile all they want as long as I get myself one of those refreshments. It is hot in this room, and I am nervous. I need to wet my whistle and calm down.

I inched towards the table, and I was noticed. I guess being husky has some drawbacks; you are noticed quite easily. The teacher/counselor/dolphin speaker announces to the room that she has a few more things to go over then we will have refreshments. I find a seat and slide down in it. I just want to be invisible. Katie is not here with me. She had to go to the room for the older Brownies. I started daydreaming. I wonder what she is doing and what kind of refreshments she will be getting. I got a pretty good look at what my group is having. It looks like Kool-Aid and some graham crackers. I know each week, a different mom is signed up to bring snacks, and I really want to know who had this week. I need to tell her graham crackers are not a good snack. While we are talking about it, a dixie cup full of Kool-Aid is not adequate. If there is a badge for snacks or refreshments, that mom has not earned it.

When our meeting was over, I flung the door open and found my mom. She was disappointed that I didn't love my first meeting. I was disappointed that Katie had better refreshments. I just want to go home, take this ridiculous dress off, and find an appropriate snack.

I am not sure how many meetings we had before a big announcement came: sleepover. Everyone was giggly and excited. A sleepover at the Brownie house. Woohoo. I was less than thrilled. I did not like staying away from home or away from Katie. I really didn't like to stay in places that had subpar refreshments. This is not going to go well for me; I feel it.

The time had come. It was sleepover night. My mom drove to the Brownie house as I cried and begged not to be left there. It was a big building on the outskirts of town. It was built like a fortress. You walked through some iron gates into a patio area. There were benches, a large fire pit, and several flowerbeds. The building went around the patio in the shape of a U. The walls facing the patio were made up of large plate glass windows.

My mom walked me through the gates and through a heavy door in the U building. I had my sleeping bag and an overnight bag. My overnight bag had a change of clothes, a toothbrush, pajamas, and some hidden snacks. I had tears in my eyes, and my stomach was rumbling. Mom gave me the talk about how this would be good for me, and I would make friends and have fun. She kissed me and turned to leave. I chased after her, and one of those ladies came over and told my mom to leave. She bent over and told me how much fun I was going to have and that I needed to be a big girl and let my mom leave. I am a big girl! I'm husky! I'm a solid 6X. I am a big girl, and I want my momma!!

I went inside the building, sat my things down, and looked around. Girls were running around, laughing, and there was one girl braiding hair in the corner. I saw large tables lined up with refreshments. Ok, maybe I will have fun. I will give it a whirl. Just like Clark Griswald said, I am going to have so much fun I'll be whistling zippiddy doo daa out of my asshole.

There were a few girls that talked to me, but not many. They would ask my name then they would giggle and walk off. I had been waiting for it to be dark because that was when we were going to make S'mores. Who cares if you have friends if you have a S'more? It did get dark, and we did make S'mores. I even had a friend. She started talking to me, and we made our S'mores together. Then we went inside and sat on the floor and started talking. I was feeling so happy that I had a friend. I had even grabbed my sleeping bag and asked if we could sleep next to each other. This is shaping up to be a good night.

What I didn't know was that several of the girls knew my home situation. It was a small town, and everyone's business got around. If your mom works at the local meat market and has a black eye, it does not go unnoticed. It was traumatizing to me to see, hear, and experience some of the things that Katie and I had saw, heard, and experienced. I never thought anyone would think it was funny. I had not done those awful things, and I did not think anyone would not like me because of them. Boy, was I wrong.

As I sat there with my new friend, 2 girls walked up to us. One asked me what my name was, and I told her. The other girl blurted out, "yeah, my mom told me what your dad does to your mom". They both laughed, turned around, and skipped back to a small group of girls. They all leaned in, got the scoop, and laughed. They pointed at me and laughed more. I had tears rolling down my face as I got up and walked toward those meanies. I wanted to tell them that I was nice. I wasn't mean. I didn't do those things to my mom, and I cried when they happened.

I never got to say those things. One of the girls yelled for her mom, one of the teacher/counselor/dolphin ladies, as I made my way to the meanie group. The lady told me to leave those girls alone and go behave. I turned and walked away. I went back to where my friend was sitting, and I sat down. She didn't speak to me; she just stood up and, moved to another spot and sat down. I made a mad dash for my overnight bag. I had tears running down my face as I grabbed my bag and dug for my snacks. I finally found my cookies and sat in the corner, crying and eating. Things couldn't possibly get worse.

With a mouth full of cookies and a face soaked in tears, I sat alone. One of the mean girls started to walk towards me. Is she going to apologize? Is she going to ask me to come join her and her friends? No, she is going to make fun of me for being a fatty and a crybaby and tell me how pathetic I am. She also has to inform me that her mom is the boss here, and I can't do anything to her. Well, I may be a fatty, and I may be a crybaby, but I have had it. I jumped up, balled my fists, and started chasing that mean girl. She could run; I'll give her that. She ran and ran, hoping to tire me out. Thankfully, I had refueled on a bag of cookies, and I was ready to go. Some of the other girls went and got her mom and told her that I was chasing her and I was going to hit her. They were wrong; I wasn't going to hit her. I was going to beat her up.

The teacher/counselor lady (no longer did she have the high pitched dolphin voice) grabbed me by the arm and told me to get myself together and behave. She said she would not tolerate this behavior form someone like me. The mean girls loved that. They cackled like the little witches they were. I walked to the back of the room and crawled on top of one of the tables. I sat there watching everyone while replaying all those mean things over in my head. The teacher/counselor lady called her other teacher/counselor friends over, and they began to talk and point. They were pointing at me, and I could hear phrases like, 'with a home life like that', 'no telling what she's been exposed to," and "you know who her dad is, right?". I could feel my face getting redder by the minute. I could feel the steam building up in my head and about to blow out of my ears. The little meanie girl walked in front of me with her crew of followers, and they laughed and laughed.

All of a sudden, I jumped up and stood on the table. My fists were balled up, tears were running down my face, and my teeth were clinched. I stood there looking at all of them and getting madder by the second. One of the ladies started to walk towards me, and that's when it happened. I lost my shit. I threw up both of my middle fingers and told them all to Fuck off. I told them that I would beat their asses because they were all motherfuckers. I said all of this as I was jumping up and down. This must be a signature move because I did the same thing well into adulthood. I can only imagine that I looked like the girl on The Exorcist when her head turned in circles, and green vomit flew out of her mouth. They definitely thought I was processed by the devil.

I stood there and cussed and screamed until I wore myself out. Then, I slowly lowered myself to the table and melted into a ball of tears. The room became empty rather quickly. Kids were ushered out of the building (I could see them staring at me through the windows), and the adults were on the phone that was at the front of the room. Ol Mother Meanie promptly walked over, grabbed my hand, and walked me to the office. She had called mom and told her that I was being kicked out of the sleepover and out of brownies. I was no longer welcome in this organization. Thank God!

She walked me to the iron gates, opened them, walked me to the curb, and then she walked back through the gates and locked them. I sat on the curb, in the dark, alone in a desolate part of town, and waited for my mom to pick me up. To this day, I hate the Brownies. I will eat Girl Scout cookies, but I always mumble, screw the Brownies, while I do.

CHAPTER 4

Our house is ready!

When my mom decided she wanted to have a house built, she did all of her research. There were several lots in town that were not in the best of neighborhoods, therefore, making them more affordable. The lot my mom chose was on a street that had much older and smaller homes on it. It was labeled a low-income area. Because my grandparents lived 2 blocks behind that street, it felt like the right spot.

I am not sure the neighbors were excited to see a new, brick home going up in their neighborhood. It was as noticeable as a turd in a punch bowl. The other homes were small homes that were at least 25 years old. For the most part, there were 2 bedrooms, 1 bath homes with a carport. None of them were brick; they had siding. Right in the middle of the street was a brick, 3 bedrooms, 2 bath home with a 1 car garage.

When we were moving in, the neighbors would stand outside in their yards and watch us, or they would peep out their windows. This was all new to me. We may have been moving into a new home, but I had never felt like I was better than anyone, and I had never been labeled as someone who was living the good life. My mom did save and buy herself that shiny, red, Cutlass, but other than that, we had hand-me downs and used things. The furniture we carried into our new home was all bought from garage sales or handed down from friends and family.

I was ready to get outside and play. Katie was busy planning out her bedroom. She knew what she had to work with, and she was in game mode to make her room her domain. I was pretty nervous about having my own room. Honestly, I was pretty nervous about being in a home by ourselves. The majority of my life was spent living with my grandparents. When we moved into the apartment, it was scary for me, but I was comforted by the fact that we had so many people so close. Now we are in a house by ourselves, and our neighbors are not sending over the welcome crew.

I decided to go outside and see if I could find a new friend. There were several kids outside playing and riding bikes. I stood in the yard and walked up and down the street. I was taking in all the new sights and trying to get a feel for my new environment. It took a little longer than I had hoped, but some kids finally rode their bikes over to the sidewalk in front of our house. They asked if I was moving in, and I replied yes. I was so excited at the thought of having friends. I just knew they would ask me to play with them. They didn't. One boy walked in front of the other kids and said, 'You're rich.' They all laughed, jumped on their bikes, and rode off. I had been called a lot of names, but I had never been called rich. I also never thought being called rich would feel so insulting. It definitely was, though.

I wanted to scream at them that I wasn't rich. We lived with my Nanny until my mom saved money to have this house built. I didn't see my mom a lot because she worked all the time. My parents were divorced, and my dad was not always nice. He was very mean to my mom and called her bad names and hit her. He went to jail a lot and had tattoos. We are not rich. To me, we are very poor. We didn't have what those other people had. We didn't have a happy little family that gathered around the dining room table and ate meals together. I had always felt like an outsider, but not because of our finances. This is all new to me, and it doesn't feel good. I don't even have a bike that I can ride down the block and flip those kids the bird.

I stomped back inside. My mom was so happy. She was unpacking things as her music was playing (Fleetwood Mac). I walked into Katie's room, and she was hanging her clothes in her closet and practically beaming. I walked into my room and looked around. I was not in a hurry, nor was I excited to decorate or unpack my things. I went to the kitchen to look around for something to eat.

My mom saw me and asked what was wrong and why I was not outside playing. I told her what happened. She told me she had worked her ass off for this house, and no one handed it to us. If they thought we were rich, so be it. Then she went on about her business. I grabbed a snack and sat down. I wanted to go back to Nanny's. I hate it here.

The next several days were all about unpacking and making this place feel like home. A pointless venture if you ask me. This place would never feel like home. Those stupid kids are still riding their bikes in front of our house and laughing. The only thing that has gone my way is the fact that Katie is scared of everything. She may hang out in her room during the day and demanded that I stay out, but when it gets dark, she is asking if I want to sleep with her. Are you kidding me? Yes, I want to sleep with you!

New things never felt exciting or good to me. Changes never felt good. A new house, a new room, my own bed, and a new neighborhood made me feel so nervous. Kids that didn't want to play with me because they thought I was some fancy Nancy felt horrible. The nights that I got to crawl into bed with my sister, close my eyes, and picture everything exactly the same as it had been weeks before, that was my peace. Then, I could wake up and go to the same school and act like nothing had changed. There were parts of my days and nights that I could trick myself into believing nothing had changed.

Up until this point, we had gone to the same school that we had always gone to. It was down the street from my Mawmaw's house. My mom would drop us off in the mornings, and we would wait until it was time for school, then walk down the street. When school was out, we would walk to Mawmaw's and stay until my mom got off work. Since moving into our new house, my dad has not been very happy. Things would never go smoothly when we were dropped off or picked up from Mawmaw's. My only saving grace during these times was that big bowl of day old bread store goodies on the counter. I could block out anything as long as I had a honey bun and a soda.

My snacking was getting worse. I had gained a lot of weight in a very short amount of time. I didn't have anyone to play with or talk to. I would grab a snack, sit in my room, and look out the window at the kids playing in front of my house. Why the hell don't they play in front of their own houses? I would get so mad watching them laugh and play. One day, I pulled my pants down and stuck my butt to the window. I mooned them. That was my way as an 8 yrs. old to say KISS MY ASS.

My dad was getting more and more angry. I didn't know why he was so mad. He sure wasn't happy about us having a new house. He knew the people that lived across the street from us. He would drive by our house or would go to their house in hopes of seeing what was going on at our house. I could have told him if he would have asked me. There was nothing going on. I didn't even have any friends that were coming over to play. Mom was at work a lot, and Katie was in her room.

Those friends of my dad's across the street were always outside drinking beer in the evenings. They would have a pretty large crowd of people in their yard most of the time. They would drink, laugh, and tell stories all night. Sometimes, they would have big fights in the street. My mom had always told me not to go outside at night and not to look out my window and watch all the things they were doing. I did. They became my friends in an odd sort of way. I learned what cars they drove and what their names were. I knew who was dating who and who was cheating on who. I could hear everything they said, and I could see most of what they did. I should not have seen or heard any of the things I did. It was not rated PG.

My dad had been calling our house over and over. My mom stopped answering the phone. I am assuming that didn't go over very well with him. He started driving up and down our street. I could hear his Good Times van roar down the road. He would yell something out his window as he passed our house. After he drove by, our phone would ring. Mom wouldn't answer, and then we could hear the van roaring down the street again. That happened for a while then it all seemed to stop as quickly as it had started. I was relieved and thought my dad had gone home and gone to bed. I didn't feel as nervous or scared. What a relief.

That feeling didn't last long. Sometime late in the night, that Good Times van came down the street, hopped the curb, and drove through our yard. It came to a stop a few inches from Katie's bedroom window. My mom grabbed us, rushed us to the living room, and threw us in the closet. My mom was on the other side of the closet door with the phone in one hand and a large cup of bleach in the other. Yep, her weapon of choice was a cup of bleach.

It seemed like we were in the closet forever. I could hear myself and Katie breathing. I could feel my heart beating in my throat. We could hear my dad revving the motor on the van. My mom had been working so hard in the yard and had just made some flowers beds that went along the front of the house. They were filled with fresh dirt and flowers. Apparently, the van was stuck in that fresh dirt. As the motor on the van revved and the tires spun out, you could hear the dirt flying. Of course, the people across the street were outside and had a front row view. I could hear them chanting my dad's name over and over, followed by laughter.

After the van drove off, my mom waited awhile before she surveyed the damage. When she realized no one was there and no one was coming back, she gave us the ok to come out of the closet. I went back to my room. I knew I would be sleeping with Katie, but I needed a few minutes to myself. I walked into my room, shut the door, and dug out my hidden snacks. Katie is yelling at me to come get in bed with her. I tell her I will be there in a minute, and I sit on the edge of my bed and look out my window. I can see my 'friends' laughing and drinking. I can hear them talking about what had just happened. I look to the far right and see the tire trudges, and I feel sadness. Sadness that my mom's pretty flowerbeds and pretty flowers are destroyed. Then I saw how close those tires came to Katie's window, and I felt angry. I feel so angry that my sister could have been hurt. I scan back to the people across the street. They see me. I feel so betrayed by them. They have seen me watching them every day. They know I am just a little girl. They know the window next to mine is Katie's. They should have done something to stop my dad. They should have done something to make sure I was ok. They should not have laughed. They should not have cheered him on. I felt betrayed, along with all the other emotions.

Katie yells at me again. I tell her I am on my way. I shove my snack in my mouth, turn around, pull my nightgown up, panties down, and stick my bare butt to the window. I mooned every single person that was watching.

CHAPTER 5

My mom decided it would be best to change our schools. We would no longer be going to the school we had always gone to. We would be enrolled in our neighborhood school. This would eliminate my mom having to drop us off and pick us up from Mawmaw's house. I knew it was for the best, but it sure did not feel like it.

I would be starting 3rd grade at a new school with new kids and new teachers. The school was one block away from Nanny's house. I was familiar with it. I had seen it all my life. It had been sitting there in front of my face all these years, and I had never paid any attention to it. It's all I can pay attention to now. I look at it and wonder what the rooms look like, what the teachers act like, and if the kids would like me. Would those jerky kids that live on my street be in my classroom? Would they tell people I was a rich kid? Would they tell people about those tire trudges that had stayed in my yard for days? Would they tell people I had stuck my naked butt to my window when they were riding their bikes? We would know soon enough as the first day of school is rapidly approaching.

The summer had gone by rather fast. I had met the little girls that lived next door to us. They were pretty, petite, girls with the whitest hair. It made them seem somewhat angelic. The oldest girl was Katie's age, and the youngest was several years younger than me. They were not allowed to play a lot, and they were never allowed to spend the night with us. They did get to play with us when they were caught up in their studies. They were Christian Scientists. I had no idea what that meant, but I did know they were called in from playing a lot to study. I asked several times what they studied. I don't remember ever getting an answer. It didn't matter to me. I was so glad to have friends, even if we were only allowed to play for short amounts of time.

Because neither of the neighbor girls were my age, I knew they would not be in my class. I had desperately hoped I could have a familiar face in my new class. We went to the school and looked at the classroom assignment that was placed on the front windows. I saw my room number, teacher's name, and a list of the kid's names that would be my new classmates. No names were familiar. Nothing was familiar. I felt so foreign.

The first day of school came. I had all my school supplies. Katie had labeled everything for me. I got new clothes and new shoes. I even had a new lunchbox with Benji on it. Katie had also labeled the inside of my lunchbox. It would appear to the average outsider that I was prepared for my first day of school. That would be a falsity. I was not prepared. I would also guess that the school was not prepared for me.

I had started complaining of not feeling well and having stomach pains. My mom assumed I was just nervous and assured me everything would be ok. The closer we got to the school, the worse I felt. When the car came to a stop, and it was time to get out, I reached over and pushed the lock down on my door. My mom tried to reassure me, that I was not going for it. The more she tried to coax me out of the car, the more I buried myself in the seat. After awhile, her mean voice came out. She told me to unlock the door and get out of the car, or she would unlock the door and get me out. She reminded me that I did not want to be dragged kicking and screaming into my new classroom.

Off I went to class. My feet felt like they were in concrete blocks. I was sweating. My head was pounding. My stomach was an inferno. Maybe I should stop and see if I have something in my lunchbox to calm this stomach pain? Too late; the bell should be ringing any minute. I swung the door open and walked in.

This classroom is not like my old classroom. The teacher is not like my old teachers. The kids are not familiar and do not speak to me. The desks are arranged in a half-moon pattern instead of in even rows. This feels like chaos. I wish my shoes made me run fast, and I would run all the way home. I know they won't because they are PayLess shoes. They weren't the name brand shoes that I had seen in the commercials that bragged about making you run faster. Now I feel stuck here. It's time for roll call, and I don't want to raise my hand and say HERE when my name is called. I want to raise my hand and scream I HATE IT HERE.

The teacher introduces herself and begins the roll call. I am feeling worse. I don't know where the bathroom is, and I don't want to ask. I am getting more and more nauseous, and I just want to go to the bathroom. I finally raise my hand and ask if I can use the restroom. The teacher points to a door at the back of the room and tells me to hurry back. I start to the bathroom and feel everyone looking at me. I knew I couldn't make it to the bathroom. I ran to the trashcan and started throwing up. What a great impression. These kids are going to love me.

From that day on, it was a fight to get me to school. Every day when I woke up, I would complain of this horrible stomach pain. By the time afternoon rolled around, I was fine. This led my mom to believe that I was faking my stomachache to get out of school. Listen, I hated everything about that school, but I really felt horrible in the mornings. I don't know why I felt better in the afternoons.

On the days that I couldn't go to school, I would go to work with my Nanny. She worked at a doctor's office. I would make a pallet in the back room while she worked. My days of missing school were racking up. I couldn't miss anymore. My mom could not miss any work. She had a strict budget. She had every dollar accounted for and could not be short one cent.

I don't recall whether Nanny was out of town or if something big was going on at her work, but I knew I couldn't go to work with her on this specific day. I was sick. My stomach was hurting. I was crying and being very dramatic about it. Mom tried and tried to get me to go to school. I wouldn't. I was sure that I was dying. The only thing my mom could do was call her manager and tell them the situation.

We arrive at mom's work. She works in a meat market at a local grocery store. It is super cold and a little gross, to be honest. I didn't care. Make me a pallet in the back and I'll gladly lay there and look at the large pieces of meat hanging from the ceiling.

That is exactly what mom did. She brought several blankets and made me a pallet. Just in case I got bored, she brought some snacks and coloring books. I should be good to go with no interruptions to her workday. She was very aggravated with me, but she bent down, kissed my forehead, and said, 'please, behave'. Famous last words.

After awhile, I started to feel better. I was bored. I didn't want to color. I kept getting up, and mom kept telling me I had to lay down. She would remind me that this was her work, and that she had a job to do. If she didn't work, she didn't get paid. If she didn't get paid, we didn't have electricity.

She begged me to behave and begged me to stay out of the way so the workday could go as usual. I went back to my pallet.

As I lay there watching my mom, I became so curious about that wrapping machine. It was a huge stainless-steel monster. Mom stood at one end and wrapped cellophane around a styrofoam plate full of meat. There was a heat pad that would seal it after she wrapped it. Then, it started its journey along a stainless steel conveyer roller. It seemed like hundreds of rollers would gently roll that newly wrapped piece of meat to an enclosed area that would stamp the price on the package. Finally, it would drop out of the other end of the enclosure into a round basket that was spinning. I watched intently. Wrap, heat, roll, stamp, and drop. Wrap, heat, roll, stamp, and drop. Wrap, heat, roll, stamp, and drop. My mom was so fast, and it seemed like the machine had a hard time keeping up. When the product that she was wrapping was done, she would stop and unload the product from the spinning basket onto a large cart. She would then push that cart out of the market, into the grocery store, and stock the meat counters.

She had just finished wrapping some meat, and the spinning basket was full. She loaded all the meat onto the cart. I watched her push her way out of the market and into the store. I really wanted to know how everything worked. It was all so shiny. I looked around. I was alone. I could hear my mom talking to a customer. I looked around again. I stood up and walked over to the machine. I looked at it. The conveyer roller was still rolling. I sat my arm on it and let it roll towards the enclosure with the stamper. I pulled my arm back and did it again. And again. I was going faster and faster. The stainless-steel rollers were whirling at warp speed. All of a sudden, my arm was flying down the rollers and then slipped and went in-between the rollers.

I tugged and tugged. I could not free my arm. I pulled. I pushed. Then I screamed. MOMMA! MOMMA! She burst through the rubber, swinging doors, and ran into the market. She saw me standing there with my arm stuck between 2 rollers. She had a few choice words as she tried to free me. She finally claimed defeat and walked into the cutting room. She asked the butchers for help. They walked in, saw me, laughed, and tried to free me.

At this point, the entire market has shut down to free me from the machine. Phone calls were being made. No one had answers other than to call the Hobart man. The machine was a Hobart machine. The Hobart representative for our area (we live in a small town) was located in a larger city 2 hours away. They made the call. He said he would be on his way, and he would have to disassemble the machine.

That was a long two hours. No one could do any work because there was a kid stuck in the machine. A complete work standstill. The one thing my mom didn't like to do was miss work. She didn't miss work, but no work was getting done. Everyone was getting paid to watch me fidget around a huge stainless-steel machine. The more I fidgeted, the more my arm would swell and turn red. I used it to my advantage because I thought if I appeared to be hurt, I wouldn't get a spanking.

The Hobart man finally arrived and started disassembling the machine. It took some time, but I was freed. I'm not sure you could call it free, though. I was in a lot of trouble. You could bet your bottom dollar I wouldn't be coming to work with my mom when I was sick, EVER, again.

CHAPTER 6

I continued to fight every morning before school. I continued to feel bad and complained of a stomachache. I did not ever have the option of missing school and going to work with my mom. I was no longer allowed to carry my blankets with me and make a pallet in the back room or in the corner. I would cry all the way to school, and I would usually end up in the nurse's office before noon.

I had not made any new friends at school. I don't think Katie had made any new friends, either. She never talked about her day, but I don't think she liked her new school. She wasn't missing school, complaining of being sick, and she had not been in a fight with any bullies that we knew of, but she just didn't seem to be thriving. Then again, it was hard for anyone to notice what was going on with Katie when I was front and center with my shenanigans.

Another school day rolled around, and another tantrum ensued. I absolutely could not go to school. I was sick. My stomach was killing me. My mom gave in and allowed me to stay home for the day. Nanny picked me up, and I went to work with her. She made me a pallet in the doctor's office. I had coloring books, snacks, a Big Red, and a strict order to behave. We all know how that goes.

I could hear people talking in the other rooms. I couldn't decipher what they were saying, but I did know they were laughing. I started drinking my Big Red and trying to hear what was going on. It was so muffled. I looked around and found a stethoscope. I held it to the wall and listened. I still couldn't make out what was being said. I thought I would hear better if I were a little higher. I grabbed a chair, scooted it across the room, against the wall, and stood on it. I placed the stethoscope on the wall. The only thing I could hear was that someone was coming! I jumped down really fast and pushed the chair back to its rightful place. I was ready for the door to open, and my Nanny's smiling face peered in and asked how I was doing. But it was just someone walking to the restroom.

All of that moving around had me feeling a little nauseous. I swigged some Big Red and hoped I would feel better. No such luck. The Big Red was bubbling in my stomach. My throat was on fire. I was sweating. I know I am not suppose to walk out of the room, but I really think I need my Nanny.

I opened the door and walked down the hall. All the doors were shut. I started opening them and peaking in. Nanny? Nanny? She wasn't in any of the rooms. I walked into one room and saw the doctor. She was talking to a lady who had 2 babies. The babies were not crying, but the lady was. The doctor told me to look at the front desk, and I should find my Nanny there. I started walking toward the front office, and my belly was churning.

I finally get to the office, and I see Nanny is talking to an older lady. When Nanny saw me, she held up a finger and told me she would be with me in a minute. I tried to tell her I didn't think I could wait. She continued to talk to the older lady. I continued to try to get her attention. Nanny had the sweetest voice. She calmly and sweetly told me she was with a patient and would be with me in a minute. I told her I felt sick. She told me to take the trash can and go back to the office; she would be in to check one in a few minutes.

I grabbed the trash can, walked down the hall and back into the doctor's office. I sat the trash can down and made my way to my pallet. Once I reached the pallet, I decided I was too nauseous to lay down. I walked to the doctor's desk and rolled the big chair backyards. I hopped on the chair and rolled myself tightly against the desk. What a messy desk! There are papers everywhere.

Then it happened. I threw up. I threw up the most forceful, projectile vomit in the history of vomit. To top it off, it was red. All the papers on the desk are covered in red sludge. It is on the wall, and, somehow, it is on the ceiling. I am crying hysterically and screaming 'NANNY'.

Nanny opened the door and saw a sight similar to the scene in Carrie. She ushered me to the bathroom, stripped me, gave me a wet surgical towel, and a trash can, and sat me on the toilet.

Then she went to clean up the carnage in the doc's office. I'm not sure how any of that day ended. The good doc gave me a shot of medicine to stop the vomiting, and I curled up on my pallet and slept.

That evening, I was fine. I was eating, drinking, laughing, and having the time of my life. It was all short lived, though. The minute it was time to get ready for school the following morning, I was sick.

I know it seems like I was faking. I know my mom thought I was faking. To be honest, there were times I wondered if I was faking. I knew I felt bad in the morning, but I felt good in the afternoon. Was it because I didn't want to go to school? Was it because Ol Bully Boy had harassed me on the walk home from school? Was it because I missed living with Nanny?

Maybe it was because I hated having my own room? Mom says we are going to find out today. She is off work, and she is getting to the bottom of this TODAY. Off we go to the doctor.

I can't remember exactly how things went or what was said. I do know they did an Xray of my stomach along with some blood tests. I remember the shocked look on my mom's face when they told her what those tests revealed. I think she thought they would tell her there was nothing wrong with me that a good whoopin' wouldn't cure. That's what people had told her my whole life. Come to think of it, I think everyone had been trying to make me better for a long time because they had all whooped me several times. Apparently, whoopin's are not the cure for intestinal blockages or ulcers. Who would've thunk it?

When we left the doctor's office, my mom set out on a mission. I'm not sure if moms worldwide take their children to churches to be prayed for or if that's just a southern thing. We went to every church of every domination. My mom kept saying she wasn't going to have her baby cut on. She needed God, Jesus, and Mother Mary to move this blockage and heal this child of God.

I was pretty stoked that I got to go to so many places and see so many churches. I wasn't really fond of people touching me, though.

Some of those people even put oil or water on their hands before they touched me. Some would hold their hand to my belly and say a quiet, soft, prayer. Others would shout and scream. I wasn't a fan of the screamers. They would tend to have tiny spit balls fly from their mouth while they were screaming and praying. I wasn't very knowledgeable on churches, preachers, prayers, or the Bible, but I did think that God probably hated spit as much as I did.

We even went to our old apartment complex to visit my Jewish friends. I loved their prayers the most. They gave me warm tea and a latke when they prayed. They didn't pray out loud. There were no words spoken. They held my hands in theirs, and closed their eyes for a few moments; then they hugged me. When we were leaving, the little Jewish woman held my face in her hands, kissed my forehead, and whispered something in a language I didn't understand. I knew whatever she had said, it went straight to God's ears. I could feel the love in her hands and in her voice.

The doctor had given my mom three days to get things moving. If there were no changes to the X-ray and I had not pooped when I had my follow up appt., he would send me to a surgeon. My mom often talked about faith and believing in miracles. I guess she wasn't willing to sit back and live off that faith when it came to her baby. Not only did I have to spend three days visiting every church in our town, having every religious person pray for me, and being added to every prayer list, far and wide, but I also had to take laxatives. I know God works in mysterious ways, but I had no idea it was laxatives!

After we had visited our last church, said our last prayer, and I had taken my last dose of laxative, we headed for the doctor's office. I was very nervous about having this Xray done. I did not want to have surgery. I was almost in panic mode about it. Sometimes when I get nervous, I have to poop...

I cannot tell you if it was God, a mother's prayers, high powered laxatives, or my nerves that were responsible for the rumblings in my gut. I can tell you that I pooped. And I pooped. And I pooped. Hallelujah. Praise be to God. The eagle has landed.

The doctor was pleased that the blockage in my intestines had moved but was still concerned about the ulcers. He gave my mom a diet for me to follow and some medicine. He told her my stomach hurt in the morning because it was empty. After I had eaten, the stomach acids had been neutralized a bit, and a coating covered my gut to protect the ulcers. All I heard was, 'YOU HAVE NO EXCUSE TO MISS SCHOOL NOW'.

CHAPTER 7

My life had drastically changed. I was taking medicine, and I was on a diet. This didn't sit well with me. I wanted to be alone with my snacks and eat myself into delirium. No such luck.

My Nanny was a nurse. She felt it was her professional and grandmotherly duty to monitor my intake. Weekends were always spent at her house. My cousins would be there, too. Nanny would run errands on Saturday, and if we were good, which we never were, we would get a treat. We always got the treat. Nanny was the story book grandma. She was a soft spoken, sweet lady. She baked homemade cakes and bought materials for any and all craft projects to keep us busy. She didn't complain when we would take her good silverware in the backyard and dig holes or drape doilies over lamps to get the perfect ambiance for a scary story or a musical. She was a little concerned when the doily caught fire, but she never had one bead of sweat on her brow. Man, she was as cool as they come.

Anywho, back to the treat situation. We would get to pick where we wanted to go. It was half of the fun of getting a treat. All of us cousins would huddle up and hash it out. We would voice our opinions and give the pros and cons of each place named. Finally, we would present our choice to Nanny like it was the winner of the Academy Awards.

That all changed after the small bowel blockage and the 2 ulcers that were found in my gut. Now, there was no huddle. There was no great debate. There was no presenting the winner. Nanny had declared that due to my health issues, we would only be going to Burger King. Burger King flame broiled their burgers, and that meant less grease and fat. I hated this decision, and I hated that my sister and my cousins hated ME for this decision. No one wants Burger King every Saturday because their dramatic and chubby cohort has ulcers. NO ONE.

As if that wasn't bad enough, I now had medication times. Just like the scene out of One Flew Over The Cuckoos Nest, I would hear the dreaded phrase, "medication time". I hated medication time.

Nanny would make me take my pills with a glass of milk. Have I mentioned that I hate milk? Well, I hate milk. Anytime I would complain of my belly hurting, I would get a glass of milk. Nanny was sure that milk would neutralize the acid in my stomach. She felt she was healing me, and I felt she was killing me.

Up until this point, I had always preferred to be at Nanny's. Now, I found myself wanting to go to MawMaw's. You see, MawMaw didn't believe in medicine or diets. She didn't even believe in going to the doctor. This was where I belonged!

When we would go to MawMaw's, she would put my medicine away and cook me whatever I wanted. She would have my PawPaw bring me whatever I wanted. She didn't drive, and he worked at his service station. Sometimes, he would be the only person at the service station, and I would declare I wanted chili. Why chili? Because I loved chili, and I couldn't have it at Nanny's. PawPaw would have to close down the entire station and go buy me some chili. God forbid, he grabs a can of chili WITH beans. He would have to turn around and go right back.

I would hear my mom call and ask if I had my medicine. Sometimes, MawMaw would lie and say yes. Other times, she would be brutally honest and say, "she don't need that ol' medicine". It became a source of strife between the two families. Normally, the bickering would bother me, but I now had honey buns to soothe my pain. Bicker away.

The downside was that when I was at home or with Nanny, they were much stricter. They knew they had to make up for the noncompliance from my time at MawMaw's. I started liking being home less. I started liking Nanny's house less.

During this time, I was undoubtedly getting a lot of attention. Katie was quieter than usual. She was always shy but was becoming more withdrawn. She started complaining of not feeling good and not wanting to go to school. Everyone assumed she was just trying to hone in on the attention I was getting. Turns out, Katie had a bully at her new school that was stealing her lunch money and her snacks. I can't stand a snack thief. I offered to hunt her down and give her a beating. Katie and my mom refused to give me the name of the bully. They knew I would march up to her and tell her a thing or two and then clobber her like any snack thief should be clobbered. I can harass Katie, but no one else can.

Eventually, we were moved back to our original school. This meant we would be dropped off at MawMaw's in the morning, walk to school, and then walk to MawMaw's after school to wait for my mom to get off work. Did I just win the lottery? I think so. I am back at my school with my friends, and I have access to unlimited snacks. Winner Winner!! Oh, and Katie is not going to be picked on any longer.

Whew, that was a long couple of months. Adios, new school. Hello, freedom. I think I might like it here.

CHAPTER 8

I finished my third grade year, and Katie finished her fifth. School is out, and summer is here. We need the break. This past year was a real humdinger. My idea of a perfect summer is laying around watching some tv with some great snacks. I find it very soothing to get the tv guide out of the Sunday paper, grab a yellow highlighter, and carefully skim the pages while highlighting all the must-see programs as I sip soda. Katie, her idea of a perfect summer is much different.

Structure brings Katie comfort. I can already see that she wants to move the living room furniture around or be the boss of someone. I say a quick prayer that I will not be the someone Katie bosses around. My prayer ends at the same time as the last bit of soda enters my straw. A loud whistle is made as I continue to suck on my straw, and I silently say, Amen.

It's the first week of summer break. We spent the week at MawMaw's house. Mom drops us off in the morning on her way to work. This is perfect for me. I can grab my soda, and snacks and curl up on the couch with a blanket. I don't even have to check the tv guide. I know the Three Stooges are on until 7 am, and then Tom and Jerry come on until 8 am. I nap after Tom and Jerry and repeat the cycle when I wake up. Katie looks rather restless and is not fond of this set up. I have heard my mom talk about trying to find a babysitter or make other arrangements, but she hasn't had any luck. Maybe my prayer is being heard because this is the perfect summer break for me.

The weekend has rolled around, and we will be spending it at Nanny's. Mom is relieved because she doesn't have to worry about getting us up, dropping us off, and picking us up, all while avoiding conflict with my dad and MawMaw. I can't lie; I am not really happy about this weekend. I have a horrible bellyache, but I do not want to tell my mom. Her and Nanny have just now relaxed a bit on the diet and medication regime.

My cousins will be spending the weekend at Nanny's also. We are all 1 year apart. Katie is the oldest, then Lacie, me, and then Stori. We all get along very well and have similar interests.

On Friday night, we usually stay up late watching tv, coloring, and being silly. Gramps is out of town for work, and Nanny is all about staying up late. She doesn't mind if we are loud or make messes. She has nerves of steel. She puts her robe on, makes a glass of Pepsi, and sits in her recliner to watch tv late into the night. We ran amuck in the rest of the house. When it was getting close to the time for us to go to sleep, we gathered up every blanket in her house and made the most gigantic pallet. It probably should have been recorded in the Guiness Book of World Records as the largest pallet because it would go from wall to wall in the living room. We would have to give Nanny the boot from her recliner because we needed to push it against the wall to give us more pallet room. She would get up, make herself a fresh Pepsi, and head down the hall to her room. I swear she was a Disney Princess. It was like she floated down the hall with a beam of sunlight from the heavens, birds chirping, and her robe flowing behind her as if it were an elegant evening gown. All the while in the other room was a loud, wild, rave of a party. Our flashlights were flickering around, making it look like a disco; our portable, battery-operated radio was blasting, and we were giggling without a worry in the world. Well, my only worry was that someone would find my stash of snacks buried at the edge of the pallet, tucked neatly under the recliner. We would finally wear ourselves out and go to sleep...or they would go to sleep, and I would sneak in one last cookie before I joined them. To this day, they have no idea how or why crumbs would end up in our pallet.

Saturday is the day we go to the grocery store with Nanny and go for a treat. Thankfully, we no longer have to go to Burger King. The king is dead, and long live the queen, Dairy Queen. Dairy Queen knows how to treat kids. They know a proper happy meal includes a delicious ice cream treat. Unlike Burger King, that gives you a jinky toy and a flimsy, gold crown.

After we get back to Nanny's and the groceries are brought in, she settles in for a nap in her recliner. This is labeled as 'quiet time'. We are supposed to find a craft, game, or activity to keep ourselves busy and quiet for an hour. Katie deems this the perfect time to play 'school'. What the heck? Didn't we just get out of school? Aren't we on a break from school? I demand a vote. I am not playing school! The vote is rigged because I am the only one that isn't afraid of Katie. I raise my hand in protest, and everyone else stares at me. Katie stares at me like she is going to make my life a living hell if I don't comply, and Lacie and Stori stare at me in fear. They are begging me with their eyes to just comply, so Katie won't make their life a living hell. The vote is 3 to 1 in favor of us playing at school. The vote is also 3 to 1 for Katie to be the schoolteacher. I have a feeling I have just been set up to be the unruly student who gets punished.

Katie sits us in our assigned seats, and she stands in front of us. She changes her voice to sound like a grown up. Or that's what she thinks. I think she just sounds like a high-pitched, bossy sister. She hands us pieces of paper ripped from coloring books and gives us instructions on our assignment. I have a feeling she is the only one having fun. Didn't I specifically pray that she wouldn't boss me around? Didn't I pray that I would get to have a summer filled with tv time and snacks? I immediately protested and said that I needed a bathroom break and a drink. The good ol schoolteacher, Mrs. Katie, has it all under control. She gives me an allotted time to go to the restroom (she even gave me a hall pass) and sets a timer. While the timer is ticking away my freedom, Katie grabs 3 small dixie cups and fills them with water. The timer goes off, and I hear her announce that my bathroom break is over. I was not actually using the bathroom. I haven't been able to poop. Remember that bellyache I had? I still have it. I have not said a word to anyone. I am not giving up Dairy Queen for Burger King. I am not going to the doctor or drinking milk. I will suffer in silence. Anywho, I returned to my assigned seat and see my cup of water and 2 crackers. I am pretty sure I hate it here.

It has been an hour. Time flies when you are having fun. Insert eyeroll. Nanny is up and doing some laundry. Obviously, God has heard my pleas for help, and Katie has decided we should all walk up to the school at the end of the street. This is THE school. The school that we had to go to when we moved into our new house. The school that had Bully Boy as a student. The school that made me so nervous I threw up in the cafeteria, library, and my homeroom. I do not want to go to that school. I do, however, want to get out of Katie's classroom.

Our field trip is now in full swing, complete with fake permission slips from our fake parents. We are all walking to the school. Katie is walking ahead of everyone. She has instructed us to hold hands and stay together. She is taking this teacher thing serious! Lacie and Stori are swinging their arms as they clasp hands, and they are singing and laughing. They are excited for this adventure. I, on the other hand, am not. I feel nervous. This school does not give me a good feeling. All of the bad things that happened to me while I was at that school are running through my head. My stomach is rumbling, and I feel nauseous.

When we get to the school, we notice that the dumpsters are overflowing with all the workbooks and blank worksheets that were not used during the school year. The teachers had been at the school clearing out their classrooms and had thrown away so much material. Katie's eyes opened wide, and her lower jaw dropped. She was amazed. She was in heaven. This was what every fake schoolteacher longed for. She could have all of these workbooks and empty worksheets to hand out to her students. There was only one problem, they were in the dumpster. A schoolteacher, especially one as prim and proper as Katie, does not dumpster dive.

My stomach is hurting, I am sweating, and I can actually hear the gurgling of my stomach at this point. I am pretty sure my stomach was screaming, 'ABORT MISSION.' However, that is not what Katie was screaming. She was ordering us to get in that dumpster and get her some teaching materials. What if I get stuck in there? What if someone walks out and catches me in there? Will I be in trouble? What if the trash truck comes, and I get dumped and crushed in the trash truck? There are so many things going through my head. I am pleading to go back to Nanny's. I think a good snack and a little time in the air-conditioned house would do us all good. My pleas fall on deaf ears.

I start jumping up and grabbing the few things that are hanging out of the side of the dumpster. I hand them to Katie, hoping this will appease her and we can go home. She looks at the papers I handed her, and you can see the wheels in her mind turning. I tell her that we have plenty of things to keep us busy for the day and we should head back. That is not what she is thinking.

She holds the papers out, looks them over, and then pulls them close to her chest. With the papers held tightly to her chest as if she were a mother swaddling a newborn, she exclaimed, 'I don't want enough to keep us busy today. I want enough to keep us busy ALL SUMMER'. What did she just say? All summer? Why would she think this would be fun? I have summer plans, and they do not include schoolwork. They really don't include schoolwork that has come out of a dumpster and handed out by the bossiest teacher in the history of teaching. I don't like it here, and I want to go back to Nanny's. I tell Katie that I am going back, my stomach hurts, and I need to go to the bathroom. That was no lie. When I get nervous, I have to poop. This field trip, dumpster diving, and the memories from this school are just enough to push my gut to the point of complete evacuation. I think my poop is so nervous it wants to leave this place just as badly as I do. No one wants to be here.

Katie is not listening to me. She isn't taking the hints of anxiety. She doesn't notice the sweat pouring down my face, hear my stomach back talking her, or even notice that I have bitten my fingernails to the numb. She does make me an offer. Get in there and get as much as you can, as quickly as you can, then we will leave. I give in. Lacie and Stori give me the ol heave ho, and off I go into the dumpster. I start grabbing things and throwing them out at warp speed. I slow down when I notice there is more in this dumpster than just paper. There is old food and other items that I can't distinguish. The further I get, the more pungent the smells become. It smells like sweat, vomit, and farts.

Cars begin to drive down the street in front of the school. Katie tells me to duck down inside the dumpster as she and my cousins hunker down behind the dumpster. I don't want to be in this dumpster at all, but I certainly don't want to be left alone in a dumpster. Katie is a bossy teacher, and sometimes she isn't the nicest sister, but she is my sense of comfort and safety. If I can’t see her or if she can't get to me if I need help, I am in panic mode. The cars drive by, and the coast is clear. I feel so horrible, and I am so nervous and scared. I just want out. I just want to leave. I just want a snack. I think a little swig of soda would really help calm my stomach.

As I am pleadingly my case, I get the signal from my gut. It’s go time. I know that I have to go to the bathroom. There is no waiting. There is no walking to Nanny’s. I started to cry. Katie starts looking around for a quick fix. She is in panic mode now. She knows she didn't see the warning signs. She knows what is about to happen.

Katie walks up to the dumpster and offers to help me out. She has found a solution. She is so good at finding solutions. It is a struggle to get out because I am crying, and sweaty, and I am not able to have full range of motion due to clenching my butt cheeks together. Finally, I am out. As I am standing there trying to get myself together, I take a deep breath and wipe my face with my shirt. Katie pointed to an empty milk crate sitting in front of the cafeteria door. She tells me it is the only solution she has for me. I will have to sit on that milk crate and poop. She, Lacie, and Stori will stand in front of me to make a human shield, and I will get to go to the bathroom without risking pooping my pants and walking to Nanny’s. At this point, I really can't object.

I fast walk (like a penguin because I'm clinching) to the milk crate, pull down my pants, and before I can even sit...the eagle has landed. My human shield is in place with their backs to me. I am feeling a huge relief. All of my stress and a weeks’ worth of binge eating at MawMaw’s are flying out of my butt. I wasn't even thinking about anything else. How could I? All of my attention had gone into sphincter control, and now it was on relief. That all ended when my human shield began making comments about the smell. Like I care if they don't like the smell. I was just in a dumpster that smelled like an inferno of sweaty farts dipped in vomit.

The deed was done. Katie handed me some papers from the dumpster to use as toilet paper. They had already been used and graded. They did not meet the standards for Katie's school and, therefore, were perfect to be used for toilet paper. I wiped the best I could, and I declared the deed done. When my human shield broke apart and turned around, they noticed that I had filled the milk crate to the very top. It was so full that the crumpled school papers that I had been using for toilet paper were just barely under the lip of the crate. They all died laughing and started talking about how they couldn't believe I had pooped in a milk crate, wiped with used school papers, and pooped enough to fill up the entire crate.

I went from a feeling of great relief to a feeling of anxiety. As they laughed and carried on, I hung my head, kicked the ground, and declared it was time to go home. Katie was determined that I would get back in that dumpster and get some more workbooks. There was practically a gold mine sitting in front of us, and she just couldn't see how we should walk off and leave it. I never wanted to come along for this field trip. I never wanted to get in a dumpster. If we back it up even further, I never wanted to play school, and I didn't want Katie to be my teacher. I certainly didn't want to poop in a milk crate or wipe my butt with a used, graded paper from some kid that went to a school that made my life hell and possibly aided in giving me two ulcers, BUT I DID. I did it. I went along with all of it. I didn't want to, and it gave me horrible anxiety, but I did it. I am drawing the line, though. I am not staying any longer. I am not getting back in that dumpster. I am not getting any more workbooks or school papers. I am not even helping carry any of that stuff back to Nanny's. Screw you guys, I am going back to Nanny's, and I am sneaking one of her Pepsi's, a snack, and I am going to sit in the air-conditioned house and enjoy a nice program on tv.

CHAPTER 9

My mom had a coworker, Barb, in the meat market that quickly became her best friend. That friendship happened while we still lived at Nanny's. After we moved into our apartment, it took on a life of its own. Those two were inseparable. If they were not together, they were on the phone. Barb had a daughter who was a year older than Katie. It was not uncommon for us to spend a Friday or Saturday night at Barb's with a babysitter.

Looking back, this is all very normal, adult behavior. At the time, it felt very abnormal and even blasphemous. That was MY mom. I needed her. I needed all of her time. She should not leave me alone with these 2 'mature' kids and a babysitter. I hated Barb at first. I hated her for taking my mom's time and attention. I hated her babysitter (probably because she spanked me), and I hated her messy house.

It did not take long until I completely fell in love with Barb. She was so patient with me and so kind. She is quite possibly the only adult in my life who never spanked me. She was also hilarious. I began to crave her attention. I guess I knew how my mom felt. It was the warmest feeling to be with someone who could make you laugh even when your world was falling apart.

Barb was a widow. Her husband had passed away at the beginning of her and mom's friendship. They both worked in the meat market at Furr's Supermarket. That is where the similarities end. Barb was not organized and did not have an immaculate house. It was normal for her to have piles of laundry in the hall and dirty dishes in the sink. The craziest thing to me was that it didn't bother her one bit. She could have a dirty house and curl up on the couch with a book and read all day. I had never seen anything like it. My mom's coping skill was to stay busy. If she wasn't at work, she was doing yard work, scrubbing baseboards or vacuuming perfectly straight lines in the carpet. I had never seen my mom curl up on the couch to read a book or even watch a program on TV.

Barb taught me to love reading. She told me it was like magic. You could travel the world and live many lives, all while sitting on your couch. Up until this point, snacks were my only comfort, and random outbursts of anger and cussing were my only means of release. I quickly picked up on the magic of books. I would read what Barb had in her pile of books in each room. I went through those books rather quickly. I started asking for books and even asking to go to the library. If you are thinking I found a new outlet, you are right. If you are thinking I was no longer hiding and binging food, you are wrong. Books and snacks go together like peanut butter and jelly.

I am a bit skeptical, as the last vacation we went on was a disaster. Katie and I had been fighting over who sat in the front seat. Katie had called shotgun and proudly sat in the front seat. I was in the back seat pouting. I can't just pout without letting people know that I am pouting, so I would loudly sigh and give the back of the seat a good kick every so often. We had stopped at a gas station, and I started in on mom. It was time to switch places. I wanted front seat time for the rest of the trip. Katie objected. mom objected. I was relentless. I wrapped my arms around my mom’s leg and wouldn't let go, all while pleading my case. She couldn't walk. She only weighed 95 pounds. I was a dead weight on her leg. She finally broke down and told Katie to switch with me. Katie was madder than a wet hen.

I kicked my shoes off when I was in the backseat. Yes, I was walking around the gas station barefoot. I hated shoes. The shoes I had with me were my red tennis shoes mom had bought for field day. They were not name brand shoes. They were from Payless. That’s what we could afford, and I should have been happy to get them, but I wasn't. I wanted the Adidas shoes that everyone else had. I couldn't run very fast, and I did not win first place, or any place for that matter, in the field day relays. I blamed it on the shoes. Anywho, I had worn them and kicked them off while I was in the car. Apparently, when Katie opened the back door to get in the backseat, they ‘accidentally’ fell out. I had no idea until we reached our destination.

My grandparents rented a cabin in New Braunfels every year. Mom had worked extra so she could take off for the weekend and afford the gas to get us there. We pulled in, and the area was buzzing with excitement. The cabins were built in a horseshoe around the river. There was a playground in the middle and several picnic tables. I jumped out of the car and ran to the playground. As I was swinging, a station wagon pulled into the cabin across from ours. They backed in, and the parents started unloading their luggage. There was a boy about my age who asked if he could go to the playground. His mother told him yes, but not for long, as they had plans and other guests that would be arriving soon. As soon as he got to the playground, I introduced myself, and we headed for the see-saw. We were having a great time. So great that I had forgotten that I was supposed to be helping unload our car. My mom walked to the car and yelled my name. I yelled back that I was playing, and she told me to get over there and help NOW. So, I did. I jumped off the see-saw and started making my way to the car. That's when I heard a loud thud and the screams of my new friend. Who knew you couldn't just jump off a see-saw and run?

My friend never came out to play again. I did see him get out of the station wagon after he returned from the hospital. He had a cast on his arm and was still crying. I feel really bad knowing he will not be able to float the river or see saw the rest of the weekend. I feel really bad, but I did not do it on purpose. Mom told me to get my shoes on and walk over to apologize to him and his family. Let me get my shoes. MY SHOES! Katie says they probably fell out at the gas station; then she smiled really big.

I can hear my mom saying she has to find the shoes because we don't have money for another pair as I snuck into the kitchen. I dug around in all the bags Nanny had brought, found some snacks and, ran outside and hid behind a big tree. It was just me and a squirrel. I shared my snacks and all my feelings with him. He didn't seem to mind.

The next morning, Katie and Lacie woke up early and went to the river. They came back and woke me up. They had found a nice pair of blue Nike's at the bottom of the river. They look almost new. Had God sent me an almost new pair of shoes because he heard me telling the squirrel that I didn't want my mom to have to buy a new pair? My red Payless shoes were not fast or popular, but they were mine, and my mom had worked hard for them. If I could just get them back, I would never complain about them again. I slid those blue Nikè's on and proudly walked the parking area like a rooster strutting. The only difference would be the squishing of water and the wet tracks I was leaving behind. That evening, my feet had a horrible rash. Athlete's Feet.

I wasn't as excited as mom and Barb about this little adventure they had planned. We were in mom's new red Cutlass Supreme. I was nervous and already anticipating some disaster. I saw a coke can in the cup holder and waited until Barb and mom were in the middle of a conversation, and I snuck the can. I took a big gulp and anticipated the burn of the bubbles going down my throat. Not what I felt. Mom and Barb both smoked cigarettes. This can was their ashtray. With a mouth full of ashes and a couple of cigarette butts, I began gagging. Mom pulled over, and I threw up.

I hate to say it, but I am ready for school to start. Ok, maybe I'm just ready to stay at home. No more trips out of town or to the dumpsters at the school. I will be entering the 4th grade this coming school year, and I think maybe it's time I became more mature. Or that's what Katie says. I think I will try to spend the rest of the summer reading. Katie has a whole series of Nancy Drew books that I can't wait to get my hands on.

Here's to hoping I can curl up with a good book, a good snack and feel the magic of Nancy Drew.

CHAPTER 10

The first day of school has rolled around, and I am not ready. I have gained a lot of weight this summer. My mom also cut all of my hair off. I had long, thick hair that went down my back and touched the top of my pants. I hated washing it, and she warned me that she would cut it off if I didn't take care of it. I hated brushing it, and I really hated washing it. I had gotten in the habit of leaning back in the bathtub and letting my hair submerge under the water and thinking that was a suitable wash job. It was not. My mom was tired of my tomfoolery. She cut my hair off. It was now barely touching my shoulders, and it emphasized my big, round cheeks.

Shopping for school clothes was a nightmare. Katie is tall and thin. She can fit into all of the clothes that are in style. She looks like one of the girls in the Tiger Beat magazines. Her hair is dark and winged back like Farrah Faucet. She has the perfect cluster of freckles across her cheeks and nose that make her look sun kissed. She is so easy to shop with and for. We literally walk in the store, she picks what she likes, tries it on, and she is smiling the biggest, toothiest smile with her loot for the day folded over her arm. We move on to me. This is where the crying begins from all of us.

Up until this summer, I did not consider myself much different than anyone else. Looking at pictures, I am not sure why kids had called me fat, other than the fact that kids can be real assholes to each other. When I entered third grade, I was 'solid'. That is the term my dad used. He would tell everyone I was tough as a boot and solid. I thought it was a compliment. I did have a little belly, and I was proud of it. I would stand with my hips pushed forward, and my belly pushed out. I did not even care if my shirt rode up and my belly was exposed.

Third grade was a rough year, and I slowly gained some weight throughout the year. When summer rolled around, I did not play outside that much. I spent a lot of time playing inside (that's where the snacks are) or reading. I had put on much more weight during the summer. I was now very aware of my weight, and I was very self-conscious. Well, I was not so self-conscious that I stopped eating snacks. I was so aware and so ashamed that I ate MORE snacks.

It was time for back-to-school shopping. Katie picked out her things, and it was a breeze. My mom was probably feeling overconfident at this point. It was now my turn. Mom would pick things out and say that they would look nice because of the waistline or that I needed to wear a 'shell' with the cute tank top that I liked. She meant well. She was not trying to hurt my feelings. She was trying to dress me in a manner that suited my body and would draw less attention to the area of my body that made me cry. I cried anyway. I cried because I had to wear husky sized clothes, I cried because I couldn't fit into the racks and racks of cute clothes for kids my age, I cried because my mom kept saying words like waistline and shell, and I cried because every time we found jeans that fit my waist they were way too long and if they were the correct length they were way too small in the waist. I cried. I threw clothes on the floor. I refused to come out of the dressing room. I screamed that I wanted to go home. Katie would come into the dressing room and, pick up clothes off the floor and hold them up like a new parent holding their newborn. She would look them over and then say things like...' this isn't cute, anyway. I know what will look really cute on you'. She would start putting outfits together and trying to boost my morale. I would be ok until I tried something on that didn't fit; then, I would start crying and screaming. I hurt Katie's feelings, and now she is crying. She doesn't cry like I cry. She doesn't open the flood gates and let the tears flow, all while sounding like a donkey from sucking wind. Perfect tears form in her eyes, and they roll down her face like little ballerinas. Her face doesn't get red. She doesn't make the donkey sounds. There is no heavy breathing, and she doesn't suck wind.

Those little tears dance down her cheeks as she tells me and mom that I have hurt her feelings and she is not helping anymore. She goes into mommy mode. She tells my mom how she should handle the situation, and she tells me what she would do if she were my parent. She ends by telling us that we are both rude as she turns abruptly and stomps away.

Mom tries to be patient, but her nerves wear thin pretty quickly. There I am, crying in the dressing room, throwing clothes and having a full on come apart, a tantrum. Mom has activated the stern voice as she holds me by both arms and looks me in the eyes. She tells me we must get some clothes and she is trying to help me. I have two choices. One, I can pick something out, or two, she will pick it out. Either way, we will be leaving the store in 15 minutes, so I had better choose and get busy and get quiet. She was not going to put up with me embarrassing her in this store for one more second. That is when I made my choice. I chose to embarrass us both. As loudly as I could, I proclaimed that my choice was to get nothing and go home because I hated her, hated Katie, hated this store, and hated all these stupid clothes. Yes, I chose to get a whooping right there in the dressing room, and I chose to be super dramatic and scream as loudly as I could that my mom was killing me. It was the early 80s, and public whoopings were very common. Several moms in the store took the opportunity to look at their kids and proclaim they were next if they acted up.

We walked out of the dressing room. I was crying and pouting. My face was red, and I'm sure my butt was redder. My mom looked like she had just been in a tussle with a rabid honey badger.

She was patting her hair down and tugging on her shirt as she walked to the cashier. She said we would take what we had, and we would come back another day to pick up some size 10 husky pants when they came in. I walked to the car, mumbling to myself, 'shell? I am not a turtle. Why would I need a shell? Who says words like a shell?'. I guess my mumbling had gotten a little loud, and my mom heard me. She asked if I needed another whooping before we got to the car. I huffed,and her response was that she was more than happy to whoop my ass in the parking lot if I thought I needed it. I loved to push the limits, but I was tapping out on the parking lot whooping.

Shopping for school supplies was much easier. Katie and I loved school supplies. The new notebooks, pens, pencils and lunch boxes. We would gather in the living room and spread out our haul for the day. We would arrange all of our writing materials in a pencil pouch or box, add our notebook paper to our 3-ring notebook and label all of our items. This was the best part. We would sit for hours arranging and labeling our stuff.

We had gone to the school a few days ago and found out what class we would be in. They post the grade, teacher's name and room number with a list of students that would be in that room. I would be staying at my home school this year, and Katie was being bussed to another school. I have a few familiar names in my class. I know them because they were in speech therapy with me. When I was in second grade, I had to be pulled from my class to go to speech therapy. I had a lisp. My teacher's name was Mrs. Gibson. How cruel is it to have a name like that and be a speech teacher? I loved Mith Gibthon, but I hated her name.

Katie and I had bunk beds in my mom's room when we were little. I was on the top bunk, and Katie was on the bottom bunk. She had gotten a coke from the kitchen and brought it into the room. Cokes were sold in glass bottles at that time. They were not thin, rinky, dink glass. They were heavy glass. The type of glass bottle that you would see people getting hit with on tv. They did not break easily. Anywho, Katie had gotten one and was on the bottom bunk with it. I asked for a little swig, and she said no. I did what any little sister would do; I stole it. I stole it, and I hung my head over the side of the top bunk and gulped it down. Katie was screaming for me not to drink her coke. She always had to throw in an insult, so she said she didn't want me putting my bad breath on or in her drink. That made me gulp faster. Katie was enraged, which was odd for her. She looked up at me with the coke bottle turned up, and she took the palm of her hand and hit it. She hit it hard. We heard a clink and saw blood. Katie had knocked my two front teeth out! They were my baby teeth, and it would be a while before the permanent teeth came in. My tongue would slip right into that opening, and I talked with a lisp. There was nothing they could do until the permanent teeth came in. I took full advantage of the lisp, though. Everywhere we would go, I would announce to everyone that I was Thadie Thue.

The first day of school rolled around, and off I went. I was not feeling super confident. I had short hair, and I was chubby. It didn't go unnoticed by the other kids or teachers. If I had one more adult tell me, 'My, haven't you gotten big' one more time, I might have a come apart. Mrs. Gibson's classroom is a few doors down from my homeroom. I am not in speech therapy anymore, but I frequently walk out of my classroom and go sit in Mrs. Gibson's speech room when I am feeling overwhelmed. She had always been so very nice to me. She would always hug me and make me feel like everything was ok. I often cried when I saw her, and she would hug me until all the tears went away.

Eventually, I was called to the office to have the talk. The talk about not leaving my classroom. I guess Mrs. Gibson had the same talk because her classroom door was now locked during classroom hours. I hate this school year. I need a snack. Luckily, when I was at Mawmaw's this morning, I packed a few extra honey buns in my lunch box.

CHAPTER 11

It is now Christmas time. My mom is very meticulous about her Christmas tree and decorations. She will spend all day and night putting the tree up. Every decoration has to be in the perfect place. She puts icicles on the tree one by one. At the time, I thought my mom had lost her mind. Looking back, I can see that she grasped to have control over anything and everything. She had been powerless and controlled for a very long time. Now, that damn Christmas tree was in her sights, and she would reign victorious.

It was mom's day off, and she had dragged all of her decorations out. She had started putting the tree up when Katie and I left for school. She was still decorating the tree when we came home from school. I guess she had gotten frustrated and moved to other things. She had a mistletoe hung up and a few other things. The jar of candy canes was sitting out, and I helped myself to several as I watched. I knew better than to ask to help. To be honest, it was just as fun to watch and eat candy canes. Maybe even more fun. My tiny little mom was flittering around, hanging things up and decorating the house while Fleetwood Mac played in the background.

She would do something, stand back, look at it, then rearrange it. The cycle would repeat.

It was now dark outside, and my mom had decided to get back to decorating the tree. Not every second of that day had been spent on decorating. Mom had to take a smoke break and call Barb. Barb was the opposite of mom. She would laugh and say, 'let the kids do it'. That's what Barb did. She let her daughter put the tree up and decorate it, or she would put it up and leave it undecorated. It was no big deal to her. It drove my mom crazy, though. They would often joke that they would swap places and decorate each other's trees. Barb would have been fine either way; mom would have had a coronary.

Katie and I had gone into our rooms. We had watched all the icicle hanging that we could tolerate. That is when we heard a ruckus. We ran into the living room, and we heard muffled screams. We looked around and saw two tiny legs sticking out from under the tree. The tree had fallen, and mom had caught it but was under it. If she let, go, it would fall, and all of her hard work would be strewn around the living room. Katie and I were not strong enough or tall enough to grab it from the top and hold it up. We ran next door and banged on the neighbor's door. The son that lived there with his parents answered the door. We told him our mom was stuck under the Christmas tree and we needed help. He came right over and held the tree while mom crawled out.

I love Christmas. I love the scent of Christmas. I love the food and snacks of Christmas. I love the music and the lights. It is my favorite time of year. But that Santa fella, I don't like him. It has always freaked me out that an old, fat man asks kids to sit on his lap. I've always been told not to talk to strangers and definitely not to sit on their lap. For some reason, this guy is the exception. I am not going for it. I think Santa is a pervert. I absolutely refuse to sit on his lap, and tell him what I want, and he promise to gift it to me if I behave. First, I am not good at behaving.

Second, I don't want him sneaking into my house.

I could never figure out how Santa got into our house. We did not have a fireplace. I always check the doors and windows before I go to bed. How is this man getting in here? I know I am supposed to go to sleep so he can come to visit, but I am not feeling safe. I will stay awake all night wondering when this creep is going to break in. If he can get in, other people can get in, too.

This doesn't feel safe at all.

Katie loves Christmas and Santa. She loves the magic of the season. She is always weary of people, and I can't for the life of me figure out why she is ok with this fat man breaking into our house. All I know, I am not sitting on that stranger's lap and whispering in his ear all the things I want. I am not going to have him tell me to be a good little girl, and he will bring me a gift. I will stay awake and try to keep him from breaking and entering. I will also eat the cookies left out for him while I stay awake. I have never been able to catch him or keep him from entering our house.

Nanny always decorates her house and bakes all sorts of goodies. She buys us Christmas crafts; and Christmas pajamas, and we watch Christmas shows/cartoons and listen to Christmas music. Nanny's house is a Christmas wonderland. She gives us the Sears catalog, pens, and paper so we can make our list. Sometimes, we even get scissors and paste so we can cut out pictures and paste them onto our Christmas list.

We always start the festivities off on Christmas Eve. We have a big, traditional meal; then we have family pictures. We have to wait until it's dark to open gifts. I think that rule was made up to give Nanny a little extra time to wrap gifts. She would sneak off to her room after family pictures, and we would hear the rustling of paper and boxes. Gramps was manning the blender, making daiquiris for the adults. Nanny always bought the plastic margarita cups, and grandaddy made us virgin drinks. We thought we were fancy. It was not uncommon to see Katie with her pinky finger held out while she sipped her virgin daiquiri. She was a real class act.

This Christmas Eve, my mom is having to work. She will miss dinner but make it in time for gifts. My Uncle is home from college. He has always been very good with Katie and me, and he has helped mom out a lot. He would rough house with us, but he also would brush and fix our hair. He was always very disciplined and very stern but fun. He was an athlete and played baseball and football for Texas Tech. His body was his temple. He was very healthy. I was not disciplined or healthy. I did not want to be, either.

I am a texture eater. Always have been. That means I am a picky eater. You wouldn't know it by my current weight, but I am. It was time for our Christmas meal, and I filled my plate with corn, mashed potatoes, ham, and rolls. My uncle looked at my plate and put a spoonful of peas in the only empty space. I was horrified and told him I would not eat those. I didn't even want the juice from them to touch my other food. He very calmly told me that I would have to eat them before I could leave the table. He went on to say that I needed a vegetable and I needed to try something that I hadn't tried. Who is this guy? Why has he desecrated my plate?

I cried and cried. It did not faze him. He stuck to his story. I was going to eat those peas. I had a total come apart. I sat there. I refused to eat a pea. Everyone had finished their food. I was still sitting there. My uncle reached over and scooped up most of the peas. He left three peas sitting on my plate. He told me when I ate those three peas, we would all leave the table. I sat there, arms crossed, lips tight. I would rather ruin Christmas than eat a pea.

Katie was nervous and tried to coach me through it. She kept telling me to hold my nose and just swallow them. When that didn't work, she tried to entice me with all the presents under the tree. Didn't work. I was hoping I could hold out until my mom walked through the door. She would let me get up. She wouldn't make me eat a pea. As I sat there, I could hear the grandfather clock chiming. I knew it wouldn't be long before my mom, my savior, walked through the door.

Everyone was finished eating, and they were excused from the table. My uncle remained at the table and tried talking me through the pea situation. He told me I would be so proud of myself for trying something new. He told me I might even like peas. I sat there. Katie would poke her head in the dining room and look at me with that look that said...please, just do it. Nope.

It was already dark. It was time to open presents, and we had not even taken family pictures yet. The other kids and adults were getting frustrated. I could hear all the complaints. My uncle became a little sterner and told me to end it. Eat one pea, and we would get up. ONE PEA. I grabbed that pea and popped it in my mouth. It was like the ball had just dropped in Times Square. The crowd went wild. The cheers and clapping rang out. My uncle smiled and said, 'see, that wasn't so bad, was it?' at the exact time that my mom walked into the dining room. I looked up at her, and I threw up. I puked up my entire meal and one tiny little pea at the Christmas table.

If it's true that you don't get gifts from Santa if you misbehave, I shouldn't have that brand new bike under the tree. But there it was in all its yellow glory. A ten speed!!! Katie, Lacie, Stori, and I all had a brand new 10 speed bike around the tree on Christmas morning. One of our presents from Nanny was a AM/FM radio that clamped on handlebars. We had opened that present the night before and did not understand why we had that type of radio. Nanny said she must have made a mistake but assured us we could still listen to music. Then we saw our bikes the next morning! Nanny quietly told us Santa must have known we needed a new bike for that radio we had gotten. How did that old codger get all of these bikes in Nanny's house? Why is no one else worried about that? One thing I do know, if he was looking forward to the fudge left out for him, he was disappointed by the empty plate. He can drink the glass of milk to get enough strength to mosey on.

We were supposed to get some snow during our Christmas break from school. The sky had looked gloomy but, so far, no snow. All of us cousins had been staying at Nanny's during our school break. We had decided to go for a bike ride. We got on our bikes and turned on our radio to the same station. The hot 100 countdown with Casey Kasem was coming on soon. Perfect riding conditions. Off we went. We tootled around the block a little and quickly got bored. We needed an adventure. Of course, everyone wanted to go to the school to ride. THE SCHOOL. The school where ol Bully Boy made my life miserable. The school where I pooped in a milk crate.

We pedaled up to the school and though the breezeways. Our radios would echo as we rode through the breezeway. We were having so much fun that we barely noticed the light snowflakes falling. Maybe we didn't notice them because the light snowflakes turned into a downfall of heavy snow in a matter of minutes. We were cold and scared. We rode into the breezeway and got off our bikes. We huddled together as the snow just kept building up higher and higher.

There was no way we could pedal through this snow. We also thought we would freeze to death if we tried. We started talking about the different ways we would die in the breezeway and wondered who would find us. When would anyone look for us?

I had a few pieces of Christmas candy in my pocket that I promptly popped into my mouth. I didn't want to die with a pocket full of perfectly good Christmas candy. We were trying to make the best of the situation and singing the songs that were on the countdown. Eye of the Tiger came on just as we started hearing a horn honking. We poked our heads out of the breezeway, and there was Nanny. She was in her little blue and silver Citation car with her hand on the horn. She saw us, pulled over, and rolled her window down to wave us over. We got in the car, and she turned the heater on high, and handed us each a hot chocolate and a blanket. While we were thawing out, she loaded the bikes in the back of the car. They wouldn't fit that well, and she didn't care. She put them in there the best she could, left the trunk open, the heater blasting, and we slowly went home. All the while, the news was breaking through on the radio, talking about the record-breaking snowfall that would later be called a blizzard.

CHAPTER 12

It is a cool fall day. The sky is cloudy, and the grass is wet from the rain early this am. The back door is open, and the cool air is creeping through the screen door as Sam Cooke is playing in the background, A Change is Gonna Come.

Suddenly, the peace is broken. There is a continuous beep from my phone notifying me of an incoming text message, and another, and another. Back to reality. Time to stop drifting off and wandering down memory lane.

I am not sure how much time has passed. I sat down to gather my thoughts about a recent doctor's appointment. The next thing I knew, I was revisiting my younger years. Why, you ask? I am approaching my 52 birthday. I have been digging deep in my heart and soul for a few years now, trying to heal some old wounds. The funny thing about age is that you really start to crave peace and a healthy soul. Oddly enough, my physical body is screaming for some peace and good health. That is where the doctor's appointment comes into play. I recently had a checkup and some labs drawn. You can imagine the shock and horror that followed when I was told my A1C was in the pre-diabetic range.

I feel like my body has betrayed me. Pre-diabetic? How did this happen? Why did this happen? That is when I sat down and started trying to figure out exactly what went wrong. Like I said, I have been on a journey of healing for a while. I have pulled out all sorts of trauma that has been locked away in the depths of my being. I have looked those traumas dead in the face, and I have clobbered them. I won't lie; it was a tussle, for sure. I never thought I would have to go toe to toe with my coping skills. I truly never thought I would have to change it. I am not sure what I am more scared of, diabetes or not being able to stow away and eat a snickers to calm my soul. Ok, ok, I am definitely more scared of not having snacks. Snacks have never let me down.

Snacks have always been there.

I sat down, grabbed a soda and a roll of Chips Ahoy cookies, and decided to unravel this whole snack situation. Yes, I said a roll of Chips Ahoy. Do not judge me, Karen. You go snort a row of coke, and I'll eat my row of Chips Ahoy. Thank God I can buy my cookies, snickers, M&M's, and honey buns at the store. I cannot imagine driving around a seedy area of town in the middle of the night, pulling up to a random person, rolling down my window, and exchanging money for my drug of choice, aka snacks. Or going to jail for buying them! Damn it, now I am being judgey. See how I justify my snack addiction?

Anywho, back to the issue at hand. How did I get into this situation? That is when I let my mind wander through the years until I came to that pivotal year. The year that I no longer found comfort solely in my mom's strength or my sister's fierce protectiveness. The year that Nanny's calm voice was not enough to calm my fears, and the long talks and gossip sessions with MawMaw were just not enough to let my mind think of anything other than the 82736 things running and bouncing through my brain like Usaine Bolt in a pinball machine. It was the year that snacks became my protection, strength, calmness, and my best friend. It was the year that set-in motion an addiction that I would still be struggling with at the age of 51.

Just for the record, I have driven around seedy areas of town and rolled up to random people to exchange money for my addiction. GIRL SCOUT COOKIES!! Sorry about the judgement, Karen. I need to clarify that I do love Girl Scout cookies but hate my time as a Brownie. I will gladly eat a box of shortbread cookies as I sit in my car with the music blasting, flip the bird, and mumble (it's hard to talk with a mouthful of shortbread cookies), 'Huck the Girl Scouths.' Again, don't judge me. I am just a girl, ok, I am just a middle-aged woman, trying to deal with the trauma's life has dealt me as I eat a snack and cuss. Those are my coping skills.

I am going to answer these text messages that keep rolling in, grab another soda, and see what snacks I have on hand. Then, and only then, will I wander through the teen years of my life.

Made in the USA
Las Vegas, NV
02 December 2025

35576334R00042